MAGIC OR MEDICINE?

DR. ROBERT BUCKMAN & KARL SABBAGH

MAGIC OR MEDICINE?

AN INVESTIGATION OF HEALING & HEALERS

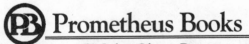 Prometheus Books

59 John Glenn Drive
Amherst, NewYork 14228-2197

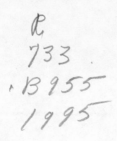

Published 1995 by Prometheus Books

99 98 97 96 95   5 4 3 2 1

Library of Congress Cataloging-in-Publication Data

Buckman, Robert.
    Magic or medicine? : an investigation of healing and healers / Robert
Buckman, Karl Sabbagh.
        p.   cm.
    Originally published: Toronto, Ont. : Key Porter Books, 1993.
    Includes bibliographical references and index.
    ISBN 0-87975-948-8
    1. Alternative medicine. 2. Healing. 3. Patients—Psychology.
I. Sabbagh, Karl. II. Title.
R733.B955   1995
610—dc20   94-42853
                                                                    CIP

Printed in the United States of America on acid-free paper.

CONTENTS

I said that the cure itself is a certain leaf, but in addition to the drug, there is a certain charm, which if someone chants when he makes use of it, the medicine altogether restores him to health, but without the charm there is no profit from the leaf.

SOCRATES

Authors' Note

This book was written by two people, and that has caused only one problem—how to tell the reader when something happened to one of the authors but not to the other. The traditional way of indicating that in the medical literature is to make a statement in the third person with the name of the involved party abbreviated in brackets, such as "one of the authors (R.B.) carries a stethoscope at work." This phrasing is not only awkward but is sometimes carried to absurd extremes as in an example quoted by Dr. Michael O'Donnell of a paper in a medical journal which read, "Since publication of this paper, one of us has died." We think that it's silly to go to those lengths to preserve formality, so we want to make it clear at the beginning of the book that one of the authors (R.B., to use the formal notation) is a doctor looking after patients every day, and the other author (K.S., if you can't work it out by yourself) is a television producer, writer and thinker. That means that when we use clinical examples in the book that come from medical practice, you can safely assume that the events happened to one of us (and we mean R.B. but we won't say so every time).

Some case histories in this book are taken from the experience of the authors; others are quoted from orthodox or alternative medical literature. When the person concerned has given her or his consent, we have used the person's real name. Occasionally, patients gave us information about themselves on the understanding that it would not be traceable to them directly, and in those cases we have disguised non-essential features (including name, home town, occupation and sometimes gender). However, in every case, the pertinent medical facts of the story are accurate and have not been altered.

We'd also like to assure all readers that, at the time of writing, as far as we know neither of us has died.

ACKNOWLEDGEMENTS

In the two and a half years that we've spent preparing this book and the television series that accompanies it, we have changed our views on a large number of issues. It's almost true to say that, like Blanche DuBois in *A Streetcar Named Desire*, we've always relied on the kindness of strangers, but in practice we've depended pretty heavily on friends as well. As a result of much intellectual pruning and preening with occasional mergers, U-turns or moments of plagiarism, we have modified a lot of the material that has finally made it into this book. Sometimes those modifications were minor, sometimes they were major revisions and occasionally we had simply to reject a previous belief or stance. Most of these changes emerged from constructive—and sometimes noisy—discussions with doctors, scientists, healers or (usually part-time) philosophers and thinkers. Some contributed new facts of which we were unaware, some helped us to defend, define or occasionally reject our own views when confronted with counter-arguments or contrary evidence. With no exceptions, we enjoyed those discussions and want to thank all the people who have donated time and mental energy to the issues at the centre of this book.

Although it is very difficult to single people out, there are some who have had profound and wide-ranging influences on the ways in which our ideas (and this book) have developed. We would particularly like to thank Dr. William Silverman for helping us understand the evolution (and limitations) of the clinical trial, Dr. Marshall Marinker for a provocative view of the way people feel ill and become patients, Dr. Bruce Pomerantz for a wonderfully illuminating discussion on the evolution and acceptance of non-Western technologies, particularly acupuncture, Ursula Wilson of Chinle, New Mexico, for a perceptive and detailed analysis of the similarities and differences between Navajo and Western-style medicine and Drs. David Spiegel and Barrie Cassileth for thoughtful and careful discussions on the interactions between mind and disease.

The television series, "Magic or Medicine?", was a co-production of Primedia Productions, Skyscraper Productions, and Cine-Media Productions, and received financial assistance from Miles Laboratories.

1. HEALING AND HEALERS

To know more about the nature of illness, about our own motives and expectations and about what it is that doctors and healers offer and achieve can only help us to make informed decisions about our own health problems.

THE WAY IT IS NOW

Around the world in every culture and in every era of every culture, people who feel ill have gone to get help from other people who they hope will make them feel better. The act of seeking help is a form of behaviour that goes back to the earliest origins of human society, and over the millennia the help that has been offered has been varied—from incantations to herbs to heart transplants. Recently, however, there has been a major change in the way patients in most Western societies seek help with their health problems.

At a time when conventional medicine continues to chalk up successes in understanding and treating a whole range of diseases, there is a constant undertone of public dissatisfaction with mainstream doctors. News stories about poor or negligent doctoring appear daily in all media, and patients are now consulting practitioners of complementary or alternative medicine in unprecedented numbers.

This is neither a good thing nor a bad thing, but it is an important change and it deserves analysis. That is what this book is about. It looks at the reasons for this large shift in public allegiance away from conventional medicine and towards complementary medicine, and at what that shift is telling us about the needs of the sick person and in particular what he or she hopes for and expects from the doctor or healer. Patients feel very strongly—pleased, disappointed or angry—about the treatment they receive, and those reactions depend directly on what the patient has been led to believe, hope for, expect or fear from the illness and from the person who offers help.

1

This book will try to avoid taking sides. It will look critically at the achievements and the deficiencies of both conventional medicine and alternative medicine and, in analyzing the strengths of both, will draw important conclusions about the relationship between someone who is ill and the person to whom he or she goes to feel better. That relationship is at the heart of all medicine, whether it is conventional or complementary, and for that reason it is the central theme of this book.

Many people may find it difficult to think freely about the major issues in this investigation. Most of us have strongly held beliefs about the experience of illness, the nature of medicine and the validity or effectiveness of the different types of treatment. Perhaps those feelings are so strong because for each of us, our bodies are the most familiar, and the most important, parts of the universe and when they go wrong, the preoccupation with feelings, sensations and outcome can be all-consuming. Personal experiences that centre on sickness, disease and illness—three terms we will explore later—therefore leave a lasting impression and generate strong opinions. Furthermore, we all know that one day we might be ill and need some help—and that also concentrates the mind wonderfully.

To know more about the nature of illness, about our own motives and expectations and about what it is that doctors and healers offer and achieve can only help us to make informed decisions about our own health problems. In that way we will stand a better chance of seeking the right sort of person for the right sort of help when we need it.

Some of the material that we discuss and examine may make some readers feel uncomfortable. Partly this is because some of what we are discussing here challenges traditions concerning health, beliefs about diseases, methods of treatment and faith in those treatments have existed in many cultures, including our own. Many of those traditions have survived because they bring comfort, even though they are not based on facts or truth. So we realize that, in undertaking this investigation, at various points we may be undermining traditional assumptions and this may prove unsettling. Even though that may happen, we feel the very process of looking at traditional assumptions has some value in itself, and when the dust settles it may allow all of us to see health issues and medical care more clearly than before.

SOME IMPORTANT DEFINITIONS

We need to start with a few definitions. The first is the word "patient." By convention we call people who feel unwell "patients" (from the Latin word *patientem* derived from *patior*, to suffer). Throughout this book, we are going to use the word simply to identify the people who feel unwell, whether or not they are consulting conventional doctors and whether or not they are called anything else ("clients," for example) by the people they are consulting. We are simply using the word as identification, without prejudgement.

As for the people to whom the patients go for assistance, there are many different terms used, some of which imply commitment to one discipline or another. Some clear ground rules are therefore needed to avoid misunderstanding. We will limit ourselves to two terms: "doctors" and "healers." By the word "doctor" we mean a person who has been through an established medical school and who has a degree in medicine recognized by her or his country as entitlement to treat sick people, and to be called "doctor of medicine." By the word "healer" we mean any person who offers help to sick people, whether trained in any branch or discipline of health care or lacking any training whatsoever. This means that all practitioners of alternative or complementary medicine—in any branch or form—are included in this definition of healers. However, so are all conventional doctors, although once equipped with white coats, diplomas and stethoscopes they may rarely think of themselves as healers—which could be an important oversight, as we shall see.

Some people use the word "therapists" for healers who practise complementary medicine; this can be somewhat confusing since the word therapist has been coined by many different specialties in conventional as well as complementary medicine. So purely from personal preference, we shall call practitioners of complementary medicine "complementary practitioners."

Which brings us to another definition, and one that is central to this book: the boundary between "conventional" and "alternative" or "complementary" forms of medicine. The exact frontier may be difficult to determine. We may, however, define conventional medicine as a body of actions and treatment that accords with the general philosophy and understanding of disease and therapy taught in established medical schools, practised by doctors and licensed and regulated by their governing authorities. This does not mean, of course, that every single action of a doctor belongs by definition to conventional medicine, since some doctors practise complementary techniques such as charismatic healing or homeopathic medicine as well as their conventional methods. Furthermore, some doctors believe they are practising conventional medicine when they are doing nothing of the sort. Every profession contains practitioners who are out of date, sloppy, biased or lazy, and uniformity—however desirable—is not possible in the real world.

Similarly, not all practices of conventional medicine share the same foundation. Although some of conventional medicine is based on scientific principles and on the results of scientific investigations in physiology, biochemistry, microbiology and so on, some is not based on science but on empiricism or on chance discoveries. Even so, most conventional medical actions do fit in with accepted views of the physical world and are consistent with the conventional understanding of the physical universe. Those phenomena that don't fit in, those that are inexplicable in the present state of knowledge, customarily become the focus of scientific research in the usually well-founded belief that a scientific explanation will be found in the future. For example, in the recent past there have been several diseases that seemed to arise inexplicably, but for which the true cause was discovered some time later. Two of these are Legionnaires' disease and AIDS—both were previously unrecorded diseases (groups of symptoms and physical problems) with no obvious cause. Legionnaires' disease was originally thought to be the result of deliberate poisoning, and AIDS was ascribed to drug abuse, side effects of seminal fluid, long-term antibiotics or a combination of several other causes, and it was only later on that the causative organisms

—the *Legionella* bacillus and the HIV virus—were identified. At the time these diseases were first described, even though the causes were undiscovered, their existence did not challenge or threaten conventional understanding of biology, physics or chemistry.

Clearly, some aspects of conventional medical practice will always be somewhat ahead of the scientific evidence, and this means that any attempt to define it will always be fuzzy at the edges.

These then are the central principles on which our definition of conventional medicine is based—however incomplete and blurred that definition may be. However, if there seem to be problems in defining conventional medicine, they are small compared to the problems of defining alternative medicine.

First, even its practitioners disagree among themselves on the most appropriate term to use—alternative or complementary? Second, the many forms of complementary or alternative medicine have nothing in common with each other apart from the fact that they set themselves aside from conventional medicine. Like a conference of nonconformist groups, they conform only in their independence from other conformity. The definition of alternative or complementary medicine is therefore based on what it isn't. Perhaps the most useful definition of alternative or complementary medicine would be: anything given to or done to a patient by a practitioner whose interventions are based on a body of consistent practices and teachings outside the limits of conventional medicine. It *isn't* conventional medicine; it's an alternative to it (according to one definition) or it's a help, an adjunct, an assistant or complementary to conventional medicine in the other definition.

But in the end, however we choose to label those classes, we are up against the inbuilt biases of language. Words are rarely neutral.

Here are some words that are sometimes applied to healing encounters:

Orthodox	Unorthodox	Fringe
Conventional	Alternative	
Established	Complementary	
Allopathic	Natural	
Proven	Unproven	

Every one of these words embodies a viewpoint. Some of the words betray the preconceptions of the people who use them, and it is not too difficult to work out the implicit value judgements that lurk behind them. "Orthodox" medicine is clearly that which is upright, correct, the right way to do things; "conventional" medicine is done the way most people would do it (implicit in this is: most people who know what they're on about); "established" medicine implies that a degree of authority has been granted to it from outside—perhaps by learned bodies or by society as a whole; "proven" therapies are those that have been put to some sort of test and passed. And if we look at the other list: "unorthodox" therapies are differentiated from the accepted methods of medical practice, rather odd and unusual ways to do things, set apart from the "right" way; "alternative" medicine is a slightly more neutral statement of the same idea—it is assumed that we all know what it is alternative to, without any implication that one is better than the other; "complementary" has the same feel to it, although in this case it is more obviously as valuable as the system it is complementary to, and implies that a wholeness or a comprehensiveness will emerge if the two are considered together.

As a working tool, these definitions of alternative and conventional medicine will at least allow us to distinguish broadly between the two areas of health philosophy; the precise and specific differences between them emerge as we go on. For convenience in this book, and to avoid the tedium of saying "alternative or complementary" all the time, we will use either one word or the other, interchangeably.

We also have to define the terms we've used in the title of this book—"magic" and "medicine." We have used those two words to reflect the view that there are two major ingredients in every interaction between a patient and a doctor or healer. One of the ingredients in the transaction is usually easy to see and to measure or analyze. It may be a pill, a herb, an operation, a manipulation or any other physical form of intervention. For the purposes of this book, we shall call this visible, material, measurable, assessable component of the transaction "medicine"—whether it is effective or ineffective and wherever it comes from.

However, almost every interaction between a patient and a healer or doctor (unless the patient is in coma) has another non-material, almost indefinable and perhaps subconscious element. This second ingredient consists of the interaction between the person of the doctor or healer and the person of the patient. That element is often shrouded in mystery and sometimes in mysticism. It also, by the way, is dismissed as of no importance by some doctors who feel that dealing with the physical complaint is the major or even sole component of the doctor's task. We shall call that non-material, invisible, inaccessible (and perhaps unmeasurable) constituent "magic." Later on we may see that some of the elements of that magic are not as mysterious as has been supposed and can be subjected to analysis and even described, studied and taught, but for the moment that hold-all word "magic" best defines a concept that is otherwise extremely difficult to define.

Finally, we have to define the terms "disease," "illness" and "sickness." By disease we mean a group of symptoms (subjective problems noted by the patient), signs (objective alterations in the body detected by an observer), or investigations (results of objective tests measured by medical devices or procedures) that are recognized by conventional medicine as having a coherent and separate existence and origin. We are therefore using the word "disease" as defined by conventional medicine.

Patients with diseases may or may not feel ill; high blood pressure, for example, may be detected by a doctor but cause no symptoms whatever that are noticed by the patient. On the other hand, patients may feel ill who have no disease that is recognized in the current state of knowledge of conventional medicine—for example, patients who (particularly in the 1970s) felt that they were "allergic to the twentieth century," a diagnosis that was controversial at the time and has almost disappeared now. So we are therefore using the word "illness" to mean the patient's *experience*, whether or not it is directly related to a disease.

In using the word "sickness," or "sick role," we are referring to the patient's social functioning, and whether the patient has decided—or is compelled—to adopt the role of a sick person in the home, at work or in any other social setting. Again, a patient may have a disease, without experiencing illness, and not adopt the role of a sick person—for example, a diabetic patient whose daily activities are not limited by treatment of symptoms. Similarly, a patient might adopt a sick role as a result of an experience of illness, but without a disease—Victorian ladies who took to their beds with neurasthenia are examples. And someone might adopt a sick role without disease or illness—as is the case of people who are pathologically worried about their future health. In some cases, that worry might be justified on medical grounds—for instance, if one parent has Huntington's disease (an irreversible degenerative disease of the nervous system producing abnormal movements, paralysis and dementia), each child has a 50 per cent chance of developing the same disease, and any worries about the future are clearly rational. On the other hand, some people have unfounded worries about cancer or venereal disease which are not based on any medical facts, but which are still severe enough to cause the person to adopt a sick role. Many of these definitions have emerged as modern anthropologists and sociologists have analyzed human behaviour in illness in different societies. But we can also learn a lot about the needs of people who are sick, ill or diseased by looking back into history at how the healer-patient relationship evolved, to discover some surprising antecedents for our modern medical system.

With all these definitions in mind, therefore, we can now look at the similarities and differences between conventional and complementary medicine—and find out what that tells us about human behaviour and people's reactions to the threat of illness.

2. THE ORIGINS OF HEALING

> *So the two schools of healing came to a parting of the ways—*
> *conventional medicine pursuing the goal of science and the mechanistic cure*
> *of the curable diseases, and complementary medicine adhering faithfully*
> *to the traditions of the healer-patient relationship.*

THE PREHISTORY OF MEDICINE

If you grow up under one particular system or culture, it's actually very difficult to imagine what life might really have been like before it, or is like outside it. It's almost impossible for urban teenagers, for example, to imagine life before the car or the telephone (or before the car-phone for that matter). In the same way, it's hard for citizens of the Western world to get an accurate impression of what life was like before the era of scientific medicine.

Yet however difficult it is for us to visualize healing in past eras, if we could go back only a century or two we would see that what we now call conventional medicine wasn't always the established (and conventional) school. Furthermore, what we now call alternative medicine wasn't the alternative to it. In the fairly recent past, the two schools were virtually indistinguishable.

What we now call conventional medicine has only recently graduated as a scientific (or partly scientific) discipline embracing a central corps of accepted philosophy, rules and regulations. Before that comparatively recent era, the ancestors of our modern conventional doctors were an ill-assorted group, comprising a few scientists, a few skilful and observant bedside physicians, and a larger motley collection of hopefuls, enthusiasts, evangelistic believers, snake-oil salesmen, mountebanks, quacks, plain frauds and con men, all of whom can trace their ancestry back beyond alchemists, herbalists, priests and nuns, to tribal shamans and magicians. The true prehistory of medicine is magic.

VERY EARLY DAYS

The earliest origins of human healing activities predate any form of man-made recorded history, so that most of what follows is necessarily conjecture (a polite word for guesswork). However, healing seems to be mentioned in the very earliest known physical records of mankind's activities—so some form of it must have been in existence by the time man began to evolve symbolic language.

In the earliest days of human society, the local wise man was probably the one who had the answers to everything. He (or probably very rarely, she) was the one who had the answers to the birth of the universe, the origins of mankind, the purpose of life and the remedy for disease. All these activities would almost certainly have been linked by a theory or legend unifying the forces of life, the purposes of the gods and nature, and the place of human beings in the overall scheme. There would have been, presumably, a sense of continuity between mankind and the other inhabitants of the planet, and a sense of overall satisfaction with the way the system operated. When things seemed to go wrong—such as storms, predation by vicious animals or occasional infections—the Wise Man would offer some explanation and some incantation or specific action to remedy the problem. If the problem was self-limiting (such as a solar eclipse), then the action—such as the South Sea Islanders' custom of banging drums and blowing trumpets to make the moon disgorge the sun—would be seen to be effective and would be repeated each time the problem arose.

Precisely what the Wise Man said we shall never know. But what the Wise Man did we can guess at. He bashed holes in his patients' skulls. Trephining (the correct term for the therapeutic ventilation of a fellow human's cranium) is offered by archaeologists as evidence of the earliest medical intervention. Skulls as old as 10,000 years have been found with unambiguous evidence that they have been trephined. The Incas of Peru were masters of the art, but the idea seems to have occurred to many different societies all over the world with little likelihood of them learning it from each other. If we are looking for evidence of the first doctor-patient relationship, this seems to be what we are seeking. And, like most doctor-patient relationships since, it was a cause of greater pain to the patient than to the doctor.

The holes in the skulls are neat and accurate, and there is usually fresh growth of bone around them, suggesting first that someone other than the owner of the skull did the trephining and second that the patient survived. So what was the purpose of the surgery? There are some clues. The holes are usually found near a pre-existing crack in the skull, which suggests an attempt to relieve the effect of a fracture. This idea is reinforced by data gathered this century from among people living in the mountains of Algeria. One anthropologist said about this widespread practice, "The native surgeons are unanimous in declaring that injuries resulting from a blow are the sole cause of the favourite operation."

Presumably the trephiner must have had some special skills—or at least a lack of squeamishness—and his professional qualifications would probably have been deduced by potential patients from the survival of a few of his earlier clients. One skull in Sardinia dating from about 1400 B.C. shows that its late owner had had four operations and had survived the first three.

Here then is the first evidence of treatment for headache, perhaps pre-dating the discovery of aspirin (originally extracted from willow bark) by five millennia or more. Whether the pre-historic healers ever said, "Make two holes in his head and call me in the morning," we shall never know, but at least we know that, at the dawn of mankind's social organization, somebody seemed to be trying to do something to heal somebody else.

EARLY MAGIC, EARLY MEDICINE

The first written evidence for a true profession of healer comes in Sumerian tablets, which were inscribed in the cuneiform alphabet in a language called Akkadian. Many thousands of these tablets have been interpreted and just a few of them deal with medical matters. For instance, what was once translated as "the sieve, the sieve, the red sieve" has recently been re-translated as "O willow, willow, dark willow." Hence it's not easy to be very precise. Even so, it does seem that even as far back as 1600 B.C. there were two types of healer— the *ashipu* or sorcerer and the *asu* or physician. One practised magic, the other practised medicine. What is more, according to Guido Majno, author of *The Healing Hand*, an extraordinary history of wounds, "The two types of healers were probably collaborators rather than competitors: the sorcerer used drugs and the physicians used magic." So the Sumerians had clearly decided the "alternative or complementary" question at a very early stage in their evolution even though, by our standards, the two sides were wearing the wrong uniforms. By and large our society tends to favour the healers having the drugs and the sorcerers having the magic, but certainly this was an early example of combining the two disciplines and is comparable to some of the other models of collaboration that we shall discuss in the last chapter.

What has come down to us about early attempts to deal with patients and their complaints is a mixture of two types of interventions. One type seemed to be following some kind of rational course but rarely achieved any good. The other—and overtly magical— kind of procedure made no pretence of addressing direct physical needs but worked either directly through the mind or spirit or indirectly through a god or gods.

One of the interesting things to observe is that the Sumerian example is typical of the way in which these two types of procedure existed side by side, and it happened in many different cultures and periods. In an Ancient Egyptian text, for example, we read one moment of bleeding being treated with an incantation, to be recited "over a Red Pearl of Cornelian placed in the anus of the man or woman." The incantation began:

> Retreat creature of Horus!
> Retreat, creature of Seth!
> Dispelled be the blood that cometh from the city of Wnw.

In another contemporary text, however, there's a set of instructions for a physician dealing with a shoulder wound:

If thou findest that his flesh has developed inflammation from the wound that is in his shoulder, while that wound is inflamed, open and its stitching loose, thou shouldst lay thy hand upon it. Shouldst thou find inflammation issuing from the mouth of his wound at thy touch, and secretions discharging therefrom are cool like *wenesh*-juice, thou shouldst say concerning him: "One having a gaping wound in his shoulder, it being inflamed and he continues to have fever from it. An ailment with which I will contend."

The physician was then supposed to contend with the ailment by using grease, honey and lint until the man recovered. The procedure of the physician "laying his hand upon the wound" might have helped by expressing pus (although it could equally well have added different bacteria to the infection) but it would almost certainly have contributed to the patient feeling better. This is one of the earliest medical textbooks to specify the use of therapeutic touch.

At this early stage in the evolution of healing, several underlying themes or principles cropped up in many different societies and cultures. They're interesting because they reflect the way humans started thinking about biology and pathology—and also because the same themes crop up in several of today's schools of complementary medicine. Perhaps there is a certain universality in the way we would like to see the world. These are some of the main themes[1]:

Continuity between man and nature

Early humans saw themselves (quite justifiably) as closely related to all other animal species. Sometimes animals were incorporated into folklore as the ancestors of mankind, sometimes as repositories of certain characteristics (wisdom, strength, love and so on). But the point is that a sense of affinity between mankind and the animal kingdom was the status quo (by and large), and this attitude persisted almost until the Victorian era. The idea that the animals were a totally different life form and inherently inferior (as opposed to merely different) was a fairly recent development, and it accounts for some of the difficulties encountered by evolutionary theorists who proposed that we all shared a common origin.

Vitalist theories

While humans identified themselves closely with other organic life forms, it was quite easy to see that something separated them (and the animals) from the various lifeless objects that littered the planet. It was also apparent that when a human (or animal) died, it became lifeless. It must have been quite difficult for early humans to deduce from first principles exactly what happens when a living being dies. The most obvious interpretation of a death is that the living animal contained some essence or spirit which left it, and the remnant, lacking life force, is therefore dead.

Not unnaturally, theories and legends were evolved, fabricated and embellished to explain the disappearance of life. So concepts of breath and spirit were established (as witness the word *animus*, which means spirit and shares a common root with words for wind and breath). In many societies, the life force was thought to be associated with blood. This is supremely logical since if you separate an animal (or a fellow human) from its blood, it dies. Hence, many healing ceremonies use the blood, say, of a large or strong animal, which might be expected to give the recipient the power of the animal's life force.

This is not the place to undertake a complete anthropological survey of mankind's symbols of health and disease, but it is interesting that vitalist hypotheses have always been—and still are—extremely popular and powerfully attractive. The Chinese concept of chi (also spelled xi) is an obvious one that has survived unaltered for millennia, and of course the religious concept of a soul is another manifestation of the same belief.

There are different degrees of believing in a physical life force. Some believe in it as an independent fluid or miasma that is so real it can be photographed (Kerlian photography today is used to photograph people's "auras" when hands or other body parts are placed in contact with a photographic plate, although a more likely explanation for the vividly coloured results is static electricity). On the other hand, some people use words like soul and spirit as metaphors for human individuality without necessarily believing in the separate extra-corporeal existence of anything physical. Even so, vitalist concepts are still very popular and there are many quite well-known conventional doctors who believe in them. In fact, one expert in palliative care recently mentioned at a lecture that she had attempted to weigh the soul of a patient by recording any change in weight at the time of death. This approach was originally explored over two centuries ago, but without reproducible success. If the soul does exist as a physical entity, we still don't know exactly how much it weighs.

From the point of view of human belief systems, then, we can see that theories about life forces began early, continue to the present day and are readily intelligible and attractive.

The doctrine of similarities

Another doctrine that emerged quite early in man's history was the doctrine of similarity. If someone develops, say, jaundice and his eyes and skin go yellow, the doctrine of similarities suggests that help might be obtained from an animal that is coloured yellow—for example, a yellow bird. Depending on the prevailing philosophy, the Wise Man would either capture a yellow bird and later sacrifice it, or let it go or in some way try to influence it to take away the patient's yellowness.

Again, this doctrine is intuitively compelling. It has a parallel of sorts in the central philosophy of contemporary homeopathy (though many homeopaths might not be flattered by the comparison) in which remedies are prescribed in small doses which in higher doses produce symptoms similar to the disease they are employed to cure. Again, there is a possible fundamental anthropological connection here—presumably we find it easy to believe in the power of a substance or an animal that seems to enshrine the symptoms or problems we're trying to fix.

Theory of contagion

Closely allied to the doctrine of similarities—which implies a magical connection between objects that share some attribute or other—

is the doctrine of contagion. This ascribes connection to or power over the whole animal (or person) to some derivative or product of the subject. Thus in some societies it is customary to heat a weapon after it has been used to wound a person, the theory being that heating a weapon that has been in contact with the victim will cause the wound that has been inflicted to become inflamed. The same idea lives on today in the practice of voodoo (among others) and presumably also underlies the fear of some tribes about having a photograph taken or giving a blood sample.

Interestingly, there was an example in recent British folklore in E.M. Forster's *Howards End*. One local belief held that pig's teeth should be implanted into the bole of a growing chestnut tree. As the tree grows up, the teeth become embedded in the bark. When the tree matures, its leaves—according the doctrine of contagion—are supposed to have the power of curing toothache.

HIPPOCRATES, ARISTOTLE AND HUMORALISM

In the early days, then, healing arose—as did magic—from legends and folklore which were at the heart of man's attempts to explain and understand the universe. In these early stages, healing was simply a matter of trying out what seemed to be appropriate—and basically it stayed that way until Hippocrates. Hippocrates was really the first systematic physician and medicine's first scientific empiricist. He travelled widely and made careful observations of human disease and the course it can take and condensed his findings into coherent and practical texts.

Several features of his work, though, tend to be overlooked. First, it isn't generally appreciated that this sort of activity—making observations, trying empirical remedies and recording the results—wasn't thought of as particularly worthy or highbrow. Hippocrates' methodology was empirical, and in the Greek view that wasn't as important an activity as thinking hard and devising an explanation of the world that was intellectually pure and satisfying. The Greek paradigm was almost a case of "I've got a brilliant theory, please don't mess it up with facts."

Second—and this is more widely appreciated but still often over-looked—Hippocrates was not simply a neutral observer of physiology and pathology. He was, as most of his contemporaries were, a subscriber to humoral theories of health and disease. Health was the result of a successful balance between the various humours (earth, fire, water and air) and disease was due to an imbalance.

Partly for those reasons, then, a lot of medical thought around the time of Hippocrates (approximately 400 B.C.) contained a close coexistence of the psychological and the physical. Amidst a lot of practical advice about dealing with injuries, we find what happened when Aesculapius's own son Machaon was injured:

> The first attentions that he received were a seat, a lot of story-telling and a cup of Pramnian wine sprinkled with goat cheese and barley meal served by a beautiful woman.

(This was clearly the inspiration for that triumph of modern architecture, design and ergonomic brilliance: the hospital cafeteria.)

In fact, the psychological impact of the physical setting on the patient's recovery was a major feature in the Greek philosophy of health. (Unfortunately, that principle seems to have been forgotten in many shabby urban family practices of this century.) Here's one description of a Greek doctor's surgery:

> The *iatreion* is roomy with "two kinds of light, the ordinary and the artificial either direct or oblique" and equipped with surgical instruments, drugs, apparatus and perhaps scrolls of medical literature. The physician himself was spotless neat and reassuring—even perfumed. He had nails that were neither longer nor shorter than his fingers. His posture in operating had to be elegant. "If he stands he should make the examination with both feet fairly level. When seated his feet should be in a vertical line straight up as regards the knees, and be brought together with a slight interval. Dress well drawn together, without creases, even and corresponding on elbows and shoulders."

The Greeks even had a type of care for people for whom all else had failed—the true antecedent of the hospice or palliative care unit. The ritual at a temple of Aesculapius would be simple: relax on the holy grounds, take in the beauty of the surroundings, listen to the hymns and wait for the night. Then each patient would be required to lie down in a sacred hall and wait for the gods to appear and give advice in a dream. Miracle cures were reported even then— one of them, engraved on a stone, reads:

> This man much suffering from a dreadful wound of his toe was laid out in the open air and he fell asleep whereupon a snake healed his wound with its tongue. When the man upon waking up found himself to be healed he said it seemed as if he had had the vision of a fair young man spreading a drug on his wound.

It is interesting that, to continue the parallels between magic and medicine, the snake is such a common theme in both. As everyone knows, the serpent twined round the staff of Aesculapius has been the internationally recognized logo of the medical profession for centuries.

However, these examples make it very clear that in the Greek model of human health, neither magic nor medicine (as we've defined them) was sufficient on its own. Each needed the other. One Hippocratic book (another textbook for physicians) states that "prayer indeed is good but while calling on the gods one must oneself lend a hand."

Although Hippocrates subscribed to the humoral theory of health and disease, his carefully collected clinical observations made him the world's first systematic and pragmatic medical empiricist. Yet, at that time, any attempt to build a hypothesis on a foundation of empirical observations was thought of as a rather unsophisticated and low-class way to proceed. In fact, there were several other major figures in Greek philosophy who were trying to systematize human biology with elegant hypotheses unsullied by actual observations or experiments. The most famous of these, of course, was Aristotle. Much contemporary Greek thought theorized that good health was possible only when there was a perfect balance of potentially antagonistic elements or humours in the body. The four humours were blood, phlegm, yellow bile and black bile, and their qualities were deemed to be hot, dry, wet and cold respectively.

Things were ticking over slowly in the Greco-Roman world. By contrast in the East, medicine was far more advanced.

In Chinese medicine—which predates Western medicine by centuries—there were five principal kinds of treatment. As listed in one of the earliest Chinese medical texts, the *Nei Ching*, they were curing the spirit (i.e., psychology or magic), diet, drugs, acupuncture and what we would now call clinical medicine (e.g., "examine and treat the bowels, the viscera, the blood and the breath").

If the order in which these methods of treatments are listed really reflects the importance given to each, then the conventional doctor is several ranks below the purveyor of spiritual care (or the psychiatrist, for that matter). But they are at least mentioned in the same breath in the writings of Confucius when he says, "A man without persistence will never make a good magician or a good physician."

At this point in the early days of medicine, there seemed to be no difficulty in combining *psyche* and *soma* in an all-embracing theory of health and disease. The basic concepts were vitalist and humoral theories, and there was a small amount of testing and experimenting going on. And while things were continuing to grow and develop in the East, in the West things virtually stopped dead. The reason things stopped had a name—Galen.

GALEN

Galen was a Greek physician who flourished in the second century A.D. and who spent 24 years in Rome, where he rose to the position of court physician to Marcus Aurelius. He wrote nearly four million words on medicine (which might have been easier at that time since he didn't have the hassle of getting articles published in reputable peer-reviewed medical journals).

There was not all that much wrong with Galen—apart from the fact that all his ideas and most of his practices were erroneous—but for some reason his works were treated as inviolable gospel. His descendants were not only discouraged from testing or improving on his ideas, they were virtually forbidden from even thinking of it. Galen's works were accepted as unchallengeable dogma for nearly 12 centuries. His thought and abilities simply made subsequent generations think that there was nothing more to be found out about human health and disease.

In fact, some of Galen's writing contained seeds of self-fulfilling prophecies that would certainly discourage acolytes from trying to improve on their elders' remedies. Here's one example:

> All who drink of this remedy recover in a short time, except those whom it does not help, who all die. Therefore it is obvious that it fails in incurable cases.

This kind of tautology —you can't help those patients whom you can't help—certainly discouraged creative research and suppressed any challenges to the Galenic model. Apart, that is, from a few brave spirits who valued scientific enquiry more than conforming to conventional wisdom.

Occasional challenges to Galenic doctrine did occur, and some of them, however ridiculed at the time, helped form the foundations of the subsequent science of medicine. Paracelsus in Switzerland performed the medical equivalent of the Lutheran challenge by burning the works of Galen. The anatomist Vesalius (1514-1564) had the temerity to dispute the Galenic theory of pores in the heart (which Galen had had to postulate to explain the movement of blood from the right side of the heart to the left). Then William Harvey (1578-1657) discovered the connection between the arterial blood supply and the veins—and in doing so proposed a model of the circulation that neatly mirrored current changes in man's understanding of the universe. Astronomy had just come to accept that the earth was not the centre of the universe but that it rotated round the sun. Harvey's theory of circulation of the blood provided a neat analogy to the new heliocentric view. The blood was the planet of the heart, and the inner universe could be seen to parallel the outer universe.

But as the science of medicine stuttered into existence with many false starts and failures, mind and body became separated. The cause of that separation was a French genius named René Descartes.

DESCARTES

Descartes (1596–1650) brought the development of medicine one giant leap forward, and at the same time set it one equally giant step back. And he achieved both with a single philosophical concept— the separation of mind and body. Before Descartes, the unified hypothesis of mind-and-body, although intuitively and spiritually attractive, made it very difficult to sort out (or experiment on) bodily problems without, as it were, trespassing on the mind and spirit. Descartes introduced the idea that the body was like a house and that the mind was like a controlling intelligence living in the attic. He freed the body from the shackles of the mind, which enabled scientists to ask pragmatic questions about bodily function and disease and thus extend scientific enquiry into the territory of human physiology and pathology.

At the same time, however, post-Cartesian medicine lost any sight of holism because it could no longer think about the mind and the body at the same time. It was partly as a result of Descartes' dualism, therefore, that we're having our current difficulties with the concepts of mind-body interactions, which is one of the reasons that complementary medicine seems so attractive.

So Descartes opened the door that allowed science into the study of human health and disease. Unfortunately study was one thing. Making people better was quite another, and for the next 300 years or so, doctors didn't get very far with that part of their job.

TREATMENT THAT DIDN'T WORK

There still wasn't a lot that doctors could actually do for most of the common illnesses. There were certain exceptions, particularly the repair of wounds and fractures. But in practice, for many centuries the people who set bones and fixed wounds weren't regarded as "proper doctors." They were almost a sub-species—superior to manual labourers, but definitely inferior to physicians.

The physicians themselves were increasing their social status and simultaneously increasing the amount of damage they could do with their treatments. Probably in deference to the humoral theory of health and disease, their treatment consisted largely of taking things out of their patients. They gave enemas and laxatives, used leeches to draw blood, cut into veins to get blood out more quickly, put vacuum cups on the skin to get more blood out that way, used sialogogues to increase saliva and expectorants and poultices to get anything they could flowing out of anywhere that it would.

Even kings were not immune to their ministrations. Here's what the royal doctors did to King Charles II when he fell into a swoon (probably a stroke) in 1685. He was attended by 14 physicians, and here is a partial list of the therapeutic interventions that they performed.

> ...the king was bled to the extent of a pint from a vein in his right arm. Next his shoulder was cut into and the incised area was supped to suck out an additional eight ounces of blood. An emetic and a purgative were administered followed by a second purgative followed by an enema containing antimony, sacred bitters, rock salt, mallow leaves, violets, beetroot, camomile flowers, fennel seed, linseed, cinnamon, cardamom seed, saphron, cochineal and aloes. The king's scalp was shaved and a blister raised. A sneezing powder of hellebore was administered. A plaster of Burgundy pitch and pigeon dung was applied to the feet. Medicaments included melon seeds, manna, slippery elm, black cherry water, lime flowers, lily of the valley, peony, lavender and dissolved pearls. As he grew worse, forty drops of extract of human skull were administered followed by a rallying dose of Raleigh's antidote. Finally bezoar stone[2] was given.

> Curiously His Majesty's strength seemed to wane after all these heroic interventions and as the end of his life seemed imminent, his doctors tried a last ditch attempt by forcing more Raleigh's mixture, pearl julep and ammonia down the dying king's throat. Further treatment was rendered more difficult by the king's death.[3]

Let's hope that future generations will deal kindly with the same kind of mistakes that we're making nowadays. Certainly some of the heroic interventions that modern medicine makes (keeping alive 800-gram neonates, mega-doses of chemotherapy with autologous bone marrow transplants for drug-resistant common cancers and so on) might one day appear as barbaric as what happened to King Charles.

TREATMENT THAT WORKED

If, as the poet Philip Larkin has postulated, sexual intercourse was invented in 1963, then modern medicine predates it by about 30 or 40 years.

Man's understanding of diseases developed intermittently from Hippocrates onwards, but the effective treatment of common conditions did not really start until the discovery of antimicrobials and antibiotics. In 1928 Alexander Fleming made the chance discovery that led to the use of the first antibiotic, penicillin. In 1932, the German biochemist Domagk prepared the first antimicrobial Prontosil (sulphanilamide), and by the end of the 1930s and into the early 1940s, the practice of medicine began to change dramatically; doctors at last had some effective methods of treating some of the common diseases. Until then, the practice of medicine was hardly further advanced than it had been in the dark ages. When Oliver Wendell Holmes (1809-1894) suggested that if the entire contents of the current pharmacopoeia were tipped into the sea it would be all the better for mankind and all the worse for the fishes, he wasn't far from the truth. But with the advances in therapy gathering momentum, things really began to change for patients with curable disease (particularly infections and heart diseases) and the people looking after them.

Think, for example, of an infection such as pneumonia or a long-term effect of rheumatic fever, deformity of the heart valves. Treating a man with pneumonia by writing out a prescription for penicillin was easier and quicker than the previous job of supporting the patient through days and weeks of illness, awaiting the crisis and then celebrating with the family if he survived, or supporting them if he did not.

The case with rheumatic heart disease was similar; the old method of looking after a patient with mitral stenosis was arduous, unrewarding and usually unsuccessful. It was emotionally and physically draining to nurse the patient through bouts of heart failure, trying (if the patient was a woman) to keep her alive during a pregnancy and then, often as not, trying to keep her comfortable as the heart finally failed. As therapy improved, diuretics made heart failure a bit more controllable. Then closed-heart surgery was invented, performed by surgeons of immense courage and speed (on patients with equal courage) using a tiny blade mounted on the little finger to prise open a shrunken valve. And more recently, with advances in anaesthetics and heart-bypass and cooling techniques, it became possible to replace the diseased valve with a prosthetic one made of plastic and metal and, even more recently, valves taken from pigs.

THE RISE OF SCIENTIFIC MEDICINE, THE FALL OF THE PATIENT

In these two straightforward examples, it's easy to see how scientific medicine produced dramatic and reproducible changes in the outlook for patients and in the work of doctors. The bedside manner, the psycho-social support, the emotional contact and the involvement with the lives of patients and families all became less necessary. Doctors now had effective therapies and their previous stock-in-trade—including placebos (medicines that have no active effects of themselves, sometimes called "dummy tablets" or "sugar pills"), counselling, wisdom and beneficence—took second place.

This tremendous change in clinical practice precipitated an equally massive upheaval in the education of doctors. They had to learn the new science, and their syllabus changed dramatically, leaving out most of the "traditional skills." This change shifted the focus of clinical care from patient-centred medicine to disease-centred medicine. It meant that students now had to learn vast tracts of science.

The change of focus from people-doctoring to scientific disease-doctoring produced some major side effects. Although the improvement in the science was a great help to those conditions that would benefit from this mechanistic approach, it had no effect at all on a wholly separate class of conditions for which patients sought the help of a healer. A large percentage of patients' visits to doctors are not for "scientifically treatable" diseases at all, but for conditions of disease caused by psycho-social or emotional factors (at least 30 per cent, perhaps up to 60 per cent of all visits). In these cases, conventional doctors search in vain for signs of the diseases that were defined and taught at medical school.

So from about the 1930s onwards, a new breed of doctors grew up keen and trained to deal with illnesses that make up only a small percentage of what comes through their door, but untrained in the traditional interpersonal skills which were wanted by the vast majority of their clientele. The result was (and still is) a rift: by the patient's standards, most of the doctors aren't very good at doctoring, and by the doctor's standards, most of the patients seem to have very low-grade, nebulous, almost non-existent illnesses. Mutual dissatisfaction began to grow. Patients began to feel that they were being abandoned if they could not come up with a genuine physical complaint to the doctor, and the fact that they were miserable was ignored by the doctor. The human element was missing from the doctor's view of the doctor-patient equation. In fact, what the patients were probably missing was the charismatic force of the healer and the magic of the consultation.

CONCLUSION: THE SCHISM

So this is how the two schools of healing came to a parting of the ways—conventional medicine pursuing the goal of science and the mechanistic cure of the curable diseases, and complementary medicine adhering faithfully to the traditions of the healer-patient relationship. Conventional doctors had become impressed and later dazzled by the advent of powerful therapeutics. It was no wonder that doctors longed for the day when every malady was as simple to treat as the acute infections. It was also no wonder that the general public should willingly join in that hope. The dawn of a real medical utopia seemed so close.

Sadly, that particular dawn has not yet arrived. The idea of "a pill for every ill" never became reality because unfortunately a large number of human ills are not treatable with pills (or surgery or radiation), but require that other part of health care—the healer. With the rise of doctor-as-technician, there was a lapse in which those in conventional medicine forgot all about the doctor-as-healer. Even in the diagnostic part of the process, the doctor became more distant and less physically involved with the patient as X-rays and scans replaced or undermined the importance of the diagnostic touching and feeling of the previous era. In therapeutics too, doctors were brought into less and less physical contact with the patients. When contact is made (as in surgery), the patient is likely to be unconscious (or partly so, anyway) and where the treatment depends on physical contact—such as physiotherapy—it is likely to be given by a trained technician rather than by the physician who ordered it. Although some procedures are given by a physician—taking fluid from the lung or abdomen, for example—often this is delegated to a junior, particularly in hospitals where isolation and depersonalization of the patient is already a problem.

Ultimately, it is reasonable to suggest that the patient became the major loser in this realignment. It was the patient who had to pay the highest price, because after the schism the patient (as a general rule) had to seek out two different types of healer to obtain the two major ingredients of care—the science (and perhaps the curing) from one, the caring from the other.

Of course there are very important exceptions. There have always been and always will be individuals who can deliver both science and humanity, and there are whole fields of conventional medicine in which patients' emotional, social and psychological factors are of prime importance; palliative care medicine is just one example. However, in broad outline, the two paths diverged and those patients who depended most heavily on conventional physicians found that their needs for hands-on healing—the sort of caring that is sometimes called "good doctoring"—were often not met.

Patients go to healers—whether the treatments work or not—because it is comforting, and because it is a socially valid thing to do. The first part is the desire for magic—and, as we've seen, conventional doctors began to lose touch with that. The second part depends on the social role of seeking help—and it also gets overlooked once patients are admitted to hospitals and isolated from their friends, family and community. The loss of both of these functions of the healer-patient consultation contributes a great deal to the contemporary patient's dissatisfaction with modern medicine.

So now we can legitimately ask what it is precisely that the patient's needs consist of. What exactly is it that human beings want from their healers and what is it that they don't get from conventional doctors when they feel threatened by illness? In other words, what are the fundamental itches which are being scratched when a patient seeks out a complementary practitioner? We shall approach that question by first looking at the consultation—the fundamental interaction between patient and healer—and analyzing its constituent parts and elements. Then in Chapter 4 we'll present an overview and a classification of healing interventions (both conventional and complementary) and in Chapters 5 and 6 we shall go on to look at the differences between the two types of medicine which in part account for the migration of patients from the conventional camp to the complementary.

3. ENCOUNTERS OF A HEALING KIND

The consultation between patient and healer contains many aspects that are subjective and are determined, not by external biological factors, but by the attitudes of the individual patient and the individual healer—attitudes that are themselves partly determined by the prevailing culture and society.

THE SPECTRUM

Despite the enormous variety of their forms and formats and their lack of any apparent common ingredient, every interaction between a patient and a healer shares a common structure. In each consultation, (1) the patient comes to the healer with an idea that something is wrong. (2) The healer then tries to find out what the cause of the problem is and (3) makes some intervention—a drug, a spell, a recommendation or something else. After the consultation, (4) the patient (or society on the patient's behalf) rewards the healer for his or her time and trouble. Finally, (5) there is some measure of the outcome of the consultation, something that wouldn't have happened if the consultation hadn't taken place. This might be a measurable improvement (or deterioration) in some physical parameter of the illness or a subjective sense of feeling better (or worse).

And that is all there is to it. In all its guises, in all cultures and in all languages, those are the basic steps in what appears to be a complex and varied first dance between patient and healer which forms the basis of the relationship between them. As a means of analyzing the patient-doctor/healer relationship in greater detail, we propose to start by examining these five components of the consultation.

The Patient Goes to the Healer

Janice Martin, a California legal secretary in her mid-thirties, had a serious accident two and a half years ago when she fell more than 30 feet from an open window. She broke her pelvis and thigh and crushed the first lumbar vertebra of her spine. She recovered after several weeks in hospital but had continuing low-back pain. Eighteen months ago, she required orthopaedic surgery to prevent future neurological damage to the spinal cord. The pain continued unabated. She says now that she has not had a single pain-free day since the accident. Conventional doctors have virtually given up the hope of relieving her pain and have now sent her to a spiritual healer. Her request to the spiritual healer is only "Can you fix my pain?"

In Santa Fe, New Mexico, a 52-year-old woman goes to a crystal therapist for "life enhancement." She feels that she doesn't have the energy she would expect from herself and wants to know if the crystals can help her.

In Euston, London, Darren, a 12-year-old boy, has been brought to the emergency department with a sudden episode of pain in the stomach. He's been slightly unwell all day and has a mild fever. The pain has now shifted to the right side of his lower abdomen. He has appendicitis and unless his appendix is taken out in a few hours, it might rupture, causing severe peritonitis.

Bill McConnell is a man of 58 who developed chest pain while walking across a square in Toronto during the winter when the temperature was -20°C. The pain didn't go away when he rested. With some difficulty, he made it to his office and called an ambulance. His only thoughts when he was taken to the emergency department were "Am I having a heart attack and if I am, will I die of it?"

Helena Ross is a woman in her mid-fifties with cancer of the ovary. Twice it has responded to conventional chemotherapy and she has been fit and active. In the last six weeks, however, the cancer has progressed again and has caused her abdomen to swell with fluid. Her doctors have told her that further chemotherapy would not be effective, and she has now come to Athens to try a serum treatment that she heard about on the news. Her request to the Greek doctor is a simple one: "Can you prolong my life?"

Dale is a 19-year-old Navajo Indian man. For the last two months, he has felt extremely lonely, as he puts it, "for no particular reason." He has come to see the local medicine man for a Navajo healing-ceremony. His request is "Can you make me feel less melancholy?"

Now even with these very different stories, it's still possible to take a very straightforward view of what's meant to happen when patients go to healers, a view that is probably held by most people. The expected sequence of events is probably this:

The patient experiences symptom X which, whether the patient knows it or not, is caused by disease Y. He visits a doctor or a healer who says, "I diagnose you as having the disease Y. I must give you remedy Z, which usually works for cases of Y. Here it is. Goodbye." The patient takes Y and usually gets better.

When the consultation follows a course that isn't as smooth as that, it might seem that the doctor has made the wrong diagnosis, or that the patient hasn't taken the medicine.

What is rarely in question in such an analysis is the existence of a fixed relationship between certain concepts—the symptom X, the disease Y and the remedy Z. We usually assume that the X is recognizable by any good doctor as symptomatic of Y and that the disease Y is some kind of external and objective entity which has, in Jonathan Miller's memorable words, "attached itself to the patient like a Triffid." And finally we assume that remedy Z will usually cure anyone who goes to the doctor with disease Y as a cause of symptom X.

But even a cursory examination of most consultations—particularly the range that we've set out above—reveals a very different picture leading to some interesting conclusions. The first is that patients vary enormously in their tolerance and stoicism. Some will continue to tolerate severe pain or weight loss, for example, and take themselves to the healer only when they are—by Western standards—extremely ill. Other patients apparently have such high standards of expectation of daily life that a relatively slight decrease in performance or quality makes them feel that there is something going on which would benefit from the attention of a healer.

The second conclusion—closely related to the first—is that somehow the threshold for visiting the healer is partly dictated by the society in which the patient and the healer live.

This leads to a further conclusion that some may find surprising, namely that the exact definition of what constitutes a disease or an illness is determined not by biology but by society. Certainly, there is a class of health problems that are seen in a similar way in all societies. For instance, if a previously fit man suddenly clutches his chest, looks white and sweaty and is acutely short of breath even at rest, then in Western society we would say that this man has probably had a heart attack, and we would prove it with ECGs and blood tests. It might be that in another society that episode is regarded as a visitation from a malevolent spirit, but even so it would be recognized as a serious, acute and unheralded problem—albeit a visitation, not a myocardial infarct.

However, not all diseases are as clear-cut as a heart attack. Some are far more difficult to define and pigeon-hole and are classified differently in different societies. In Germany, for example, doctors prescribe six times the amount of heart drugs per person than in England or France.[1] This is not because of a greater incidence of coronary artery disease in Germany—in fact, there is less of it than in France—and it clearly has no effect on death rates since the mortality from all forms of heart disease is the same in all countries. One of the major reasons is that the German language doesn't have a way of distinguishing heart problems from any other kind of chest pain. The word *Herzinsuffizienz* is used to describe a wide range of different types of chest pain. It is probably best translated as "heart insufficiency" but is commonly used as a diagnosis without any corroborating evidence of actual heart disease.

In fact, there isn't a really accurate English translation precisely because the English and the Americans don't attribute vague chest pains to the heart unless there's some solid evidence for genuine heart disease. Thus *Herzinsuffizienz* is an illness-label that is almost exclusive to Germany—hence, perhaps, the excessive prescription of heart drugs.

In the same way, in France, a large number of non-specific symptoms are attributed to a *crise de foie*—a "crisis of the liver." In fact, approximately 80 per cent of problems attributed to a crisis of the liver are actually migraine. And most of the rest are minor gastrointestinal conditions.[2] Thus the French define their minor illnesses in a particular way which contrasts sharply with the situation in England, where the liver is taken very seriously, especially when it goes wrong.

Another demonstration of the social definition of illness can be seen in the different ways in which doctors assess the psychiatric problems of their patients. English psychiatrists tend to over-report symptoms that are more florid than normal and tend to under-report signs of under-activity. Thus one group of English psychiatrists diagnosed manic-depressive illness in 23 per cent of a group of patients while the French figure was 5 per cent. The West Germans were in between with 14 per cent.[3]

Similarly, in the American medical view, minor illnesses are much more likely to be ascribed to (unspecified) viral illnesses. This is in line with the prevailing mood of the times in America in which disease is seen as an external invasive threat and there is a predilection for diagnosing infections since they can often be dealt with actively and quickly.

Even the interpretation of something as apparently objective as blood pressure can be subject to cultural influence. For instance, a systolic blood pressure of 100 mmHg—the normal being 120—is regarded as a disease in France but as a normal variant in Britain and the United States.

So what then is an illness and what is a disease—and where are their boundaries? Perhaps the fundamental distinguishing feature is that both illnesses and diseases are events that should not happen in the normal run of life's events. A disease is something caused by a recognized organic process, and an illness is a set of symptoms (with or without an underlying disease process) that the prevailing society and culture accept as outside the normal range of everyday life.

Now consider a common event (in many lives)—a hangover. We all expect a hangover if we drink excessively; so is a hangover an expected consequence of ordinary life or is it a disease? Whether or not it is a disease, is it an illness? What about bereavement? We expect to be sad after the death of someone we love—if the bereaved person cries continuously for a week, is that an illness? If he or she cries for six months, is that an illness? And what about adolescence? In Montana, a change in financing of private hospitals led to many general hospitals quickly changing themselves into psychiatric hospitals. Unfortunately, there were not enough patients to fill them, so there was a sudden epidemic of new diagnoses. Teenagers who had falling grades at school were now diagnosed as psychiatrically disturbed (with a major advertising campaign to get the point across to the parents) and were admitted to hospital—at four times the rate that occurred in neighbouring Utah. Adolescence was clearly a disease in Montana. Is it a disease in Utah or anywhere else, and, if so, is it being under-diagnosed everywhere except Montana?

These questions again emphasize the partly arbitrary—and rather parochial—definitions of disease and illness. Each society decides for itself at the time what are legitimately regarded as diseases or illnesses. Those definitions vary from culture to culture. Furthermore, those conditions that we regard as normal today may be diagnosed as illnesses tomorrow.

For instance, suppose that a hard-working professional person (a doctor, say, to select an example purely at random) happens to get home after a long arduous day and is snappish and short-tempered with everybody. In current terms we would say that this person was merely bad-tempered and irritable after a long day. Perhaps in 30 years' time, however, researchers in neuro-biochemistry will demonstrate that this state is due to a deficiency of the neurotransmitter (brain-chemical) *gamma-tendalovin*, which modulates a soothing, low-frequency brainwave throughout the brain stem, because all the reserves of that chemical were used up during the working day. The person will then be given a prescription for two tablets of *gamma-tendalovin* each evening on bad days, following which—as if by magic—there will be no more end-of-the-day irritability and bad temper. Evening snappishness will have become a disease (*gamma-tendalovin* deficiency or, more correctly, *hypo-gamma-tendalovinaemia*) with its own specific symptoms (i.e., illness) and will have its specific remedy.

In each of the examples that we presented at the beginning of this section, the patient has reached the same conclusion: "The way I feel now is worse than I would expect from the ups and downs of normal life—it's time for me to see a healer."

This then is the start of the patient-healer consultation, and we suggest that this event is defined not by the disease or the treatment, but by that society's definition of illnesses and by the patient's own assessment of his or her state in relation to that definition. Hence even the beginning of the doctor-healer relationship is loaded with social factors, presuppositions and expectations.

THE DIAGNOSIS

Once the patient comes in and says his or her piece—or even before the patient has begun to speak—the healer makes an assessment of the situation, trying to reach a diagnosis of what is causing the patient's problem.

Janice, the young legal secretary who broke her back falling from an open window, lies down on the spiritual healer's couch with great difficulty. The spiritual healer bends over her, moving her hands up and down over Janice's spine. After a few moments, the healer closes her eyes and starts breathing heavily. She becomes visibly excited. "I feel a cold spot...There's a cold spot here...Now I'm burning up...I'm like a boiler." She diagnoses a blockage in the flow of energy in the middle of Janice's back, at the upper level of the area in which Janice feels the back pain. She has found the problem—the energy flow is obstructed, and Janice's spine is cold below the blockage.

Bill McConnell, the man with angina, has an ECG. It shows that his heart is under strain. Samples of his blood are tested for certain enzymes that are released from damaged heart muscles. These tests are negative, showing that Bill has not had a heart attack. The next day, under local anaesthetic, Bill has a coronary angiogram, in which a slender plastic tube (a catheter) is pushed up an artery in his leg into the coronary arteries of the heart. Injection of dye into the arteries shows that one of the coronary arteries is 60 per cent blocked. A diagnosis has been made: Bill has coronary insufficiency.

Darren is the 12-year-old boy in Euston, London, with pain in the right side of the abdomen. The doctor has made a provisional diagnosis of acute appendicitis and has taken a full-blood count (to look for evidence of infection) and asked for a quick test of Darren's urine to make sure this isn't a urinary infection masquerading as acute appendicitis. The urine test is clear. The white cell count in the blood is 16.2 (the upper limit of normal being about 10). The diagnosis is confirmed, and the anaesthetist is called.

As with the problems that make people seek healing in the first place, we can find some fundamental resemblances between the sort of things different types of healers do to their patients in the process of making a diagnosis.

In each instance, an expert scrutinizes something that is often unintelligible to the patient—a high white cell count, a silhouette on an X-ray image-intensifier—and says (or implies), "I have seen many things of this sort. In my experience what I have found here suggests that in this particular case the problem is due to the appendix/blockage of energy flow/disturbance of the spirit."

It might seem to many of us that this is something that can easily be tested and proven (or disproven). It would appear that the skill and accuracy of the diagnostician is a simple matter to test: either the healer is right, or else he or she is wrong. If the healer is right, then that particular diagnostic method is clearly accurate (at least in this case); if not then perhaps the method is ineffective, or the healer is not as good a diagnostician as he or she hoped. On the other hand, this may be one of the cases where a highly effective method does not happen to work, after all, X-rays and scans do not give a clear-cut answer in every single case, so why should anything else?

However, there is much more to this process than its appearance suggests.

To begin with, a diagnostician may make a pronouncement that is simply untestable and unprovable. In conventional medicine nowadays, this is relatively rare. If a female patient has a mass in the pelvis, for example, it may not be clear immediately after examination of the pelvis whether the mass is simply a fibroid (a common and totally benign tumour of the womb) or a cyst on an ovary. Faced with this difficulty, the patient's doctor is likely to order an ultrasound test. The ultrasound has a 90 per cent chance of distinguishing between a fibroid and an ovarian cyst. In other words, the test yields the correct answer 90 times out of 100. That fact has been established by comparing the results of the ultrasound to the findings following surgery on the same patients. The ultrasound test has been validated against surgery, and the results are available to anyone who wants to look them up in the medical journals.

Sometimes, a description of how to use a diagnostic method may be phrased in such a vague way that it is simply untestable. If the charismatic healer says, "Your aura is weak over your right shoulder," it may not be possible to prove or disprove that conclusion. If the patient says that there does not seem to be anything wrong in the area of the right shoulder, the healer may reply that the weakness of the aura in that area simply signifies a problem somewhere in the body that may make itself known at some time in the future and not necessarily in the shoulder itself. Such a statement made by a healer (and this is not an uncommon form of response) is untestable.

In many other cases, however, the diagnosis can be *tested* and confirmed (or disproved). Even then, there may be more to the diagnostic process than the overt act carried out by the diagnostician. If, for instance, a healer makes a correct diagnosis using aura healing or crystal selection, he or she may be utilizing more methods than appearances would suggest.

Basically, all healers when they make a diagnosis are doing more than they seem to be and may even be doing more than they think they are or believe they are. There are a large number of general signs of illness that almost anyone can detect with a little experience. The patient's complexion may be very pale (suggesting anaemia); there may have been recent weight loss (the cheeks are sunken, the shirt collar is loose); the patient may move slowly with pain (suggesting arthritis or back troubles) or breathlessness (suggesting lung disease); the patient may look worried or anxious—and so on.

At a more advanced level, there are hundreds of what are called in conventional medicine "general physical signs"—changes in the body that the healer can observe (without doing anything to the patient) which reveal disease or problems elsewhere in the body. An obvious example is jaundice; when the outflow of bile from the liver is blocked, the bile accumulates in the liver, spills over into the blood and makes the sclerae (the whites of the eyes) go yellow. Similarly, when the lungs are not working well, the blood going through them does not turn from blue to the normal pink, but stays partly blue; this can be seen in the lips, the tongue and the nailbeds. There are many others signs—the bulging eyes of thyroid over-activity, the tremor and rigidity of Parkinson's disease, the bent and swollen knuckles of rheumatoid arthritis, the knobbly joints of osteoarthritis, the clubbed fingernails of lung disease, the smooth tongue of vitamin deficiency, the pulsing neck veins of heart problems, the enlarged jaw of over-secretion of growth hormone and so on. All these observations have been tested over the years by looking for these physical signs in patients who are known to have the disease concerned, or by means of surgery or (particularly a few decades ago) post mortem examinations.

At a more mundane level, these general physical signs of underlying disease are deemed so important to the clinical skills of a doctor that they make up a part of the higher examinations of doctors in Britain. A doctor in training will be conducted along a row of volunteer patients who are asked by the examiners to show one part of the body—the hands or the face or the knee—and the student will be required to make an instant diagnosis without asking any questions or touching the patient. This is not intended to test any magical or mystical powers that the student might possess; it is simply to test her or his ability to remember and use all these observations that he had been shown during the years of medical training.

Obviously not every practitioner of complementary medicine has had seven years of medical school training. Yet even without any formal training and with only the accumulated experience of seeing a long succession of people in healer-patient encounters, the healer may still recognize that blue lips mean the patient will probably have some breathlessness, that very pale skin means tiredness and lack of energy and so on, even though he may not be aware of the reason the blood becomes blue.

The point here may appear to be a minor one, but it is very important. A Chinese doctor takes the pulse with three fingers at three different levels at each wrist. Thus, he or she takes a fingertip picture of the pulse from 18 different angles. The Chinese physicians describe the pulse in ways that would totally baffle a Western physician. Some of the phrases used in traditional Chinese medicine to describe the pulse include sharp as a hook, fine as a hair, taut as a music string, dead as a rock, smooth as a flowing stream, continuous like a string of pearls, slightly indented in the middle, the front crooked and the back delayed, soft and fluttering like floating feathers blown by the wind, elastic like a bending pole, taut as a bow when first bent, following up delicately like a cock treading ground or lifting a foot, sharp as a bird's beak, like water dripping through the roof, resonant like striking a stone, rapid as the edge of a knife in cutting, vibrating as when one stops the strings of a musical instrument, light as flicking the skin with a plume, arriving like a suspended hook, multiple as the seeds of the flower blossom, like burning firewood, like leaves scattering, like visiting strangers, like a dry mudball, like mixing lacquer, like spring water welling up, like sparse earth, like being stopped by a horizontal partition, like a suspended curtain, like a sword lying flat ready to be used, like a smooth pill, like glory.[4]

Chinese physicians claim that they can detect diseases in specific organs such as the liver or the stomach or the "triple heater" (a major component of the chi system and a concept for which there is no equivalent in Western medicine). Now, the Chinese doctor is almost certainly a more skilled pulse-taker than a Western-trained physician (who might note in more prosaic terms the rate, regularity, volume and type of rise and fall of the pulse wave). However, that does not necessarily mean that the Chinese physician is basing the diagnosis on the pulse alone. While taking the pulse, the doctor looks at the patient, the facial expression, the rate of breathing, the eyes and so on—and, if the physician is experienced, the information gained from these other observations will add to (or refute) the information picked up from the pulse.

This sort of knowledge can be gleaned almost subconsciously, so that when a healer comes up with a diagnosis that turns out to be correct, he may really believe that it has arisen from the system he is using, rather than through more conventional means. If you make a pendulum (a small key on the end of a piece of string will do), it can be used to confirm the sex of a human or animal. Ask someone to hold out his or her hand and hold the pendulum as steadily as you can over it. If the person is male, the pendulum will move in a straight line backwards and forwards. If she is female, it will describe a circle. What link can there be between someone's sex and the movement in a gravitational field of a few grams of metal under tension? The link is the connection between your brain cells and tiny muscles in your fingertips that are holding the string. Without any conscious effort, your fingertip muscles can twitch to make the string move in a circle and twitch differently to make it move in a straight line.

If we had said that the pendulum moved in a *circle* for males and a *straight line* for females, that is how it would have moved, because the movement is derived entirely from your knowledge (or belief) about what was meant to happen.

What this means for alternative medicine is that the methods of diagnosis that a healer uses may have nothing to do with the accuracy of the diagnosis. If it is accurate, that accuracy may have nothing to do with the indicators the healer thinks he is using, such as dowsing rods, pendulums, patterns in the iris (see below), auras around the patient and other alternative diagnostic aids. Rather, it is because the healer has acquired the knowledge that enables him to diagnose correctly in the same way as a doctor.

The pendulum demonstration shows that our knowledge can

influence our actions entirely unconsciously and that it is not an accusation of fraud to say of a particular healer that his diagnostic successes are nothing to do with his particular system of diagnosis.

A complementary system of diagnosis: iridology

Most complementary therapies derive their methodology from a complete system in which the diagnosis of disease and the treatment of it are based on the same fundamental understanding of human biology and pathology. Interestingly, though, there is one system of complementary medicine that has only the diagnostic component. It is called iridology and it has a great many adherents (and practitioners). It is worth spending a little time on the subject, because it is an excellent example of the central differences between conventional and complementary medicine and the way in which each looks for evidence of disease and evaluates the results of its methods.

> Louisa Lyons consulted an iridologist because she had been suffering from severe stomach pains, indigestion and aches and pains in her arms, neck and head. Several visits to a conventional doctor and a couple of hospital investigations had failed to show the cause, and when the doctors suggested a colonoscopy (the examination of the colon with a long flexible lighted tube), Linda refused. The iridologist looked carefully at Linda's irises, and on the basis of the way they looked, she diagnosed a large bowel pocket in the splenic area, stomach acidity, hyperactive autonomic nervous system and inactive lymphatic system.

Perhaps that sounds a little bizarre—but that may be because the discipline of iridology is based on a most peculiar incident in the last century. In 1836, a ten-year-old Hungarian boy, Ignatz von Peczely, accidentally broke the leg of an owl. He then noticed that the iris of one of the owl's eyes had a single sharp black line in it. Von Peczely nursed the owl until the leg was mended, at which point he noted that the line in the iris had disappeared. With a display of precocity never equalled in the history of medicine, he concluded that there was a causal relationship between the fracture and the iris line and hypothesized that the entire body was represented in the iris, each part of the body being associated with a specific area of the iris. When in later life he became a doctor, he constructed charts of the iris (left and right) showing these associations. Iridology flourished in the middle of the nineteenth century and was extremely popular in various parts of Europe. However, it gradually fell into disuse (and perhaps disrepute) until its recent come-back in the early 1970s. It is now practised in many Western societies, usually in large cities, and its clientele tend to be from among the educated and middle-class sections of society.

As a diagnostic method, iridology has a large number of adherents, but, as we've just seen, this does not mean that it is necessarily valid. Iridologists can be perceptive individuals with good clinical skills, even if they are not aware of them. Contact with the patient *is* an essential component of their diagnostic process. In fact, a careful study from San Diego demonstrated this—when shown photographs of 143 irises without ever meeting the patients, the iridologists did no better than chance in making the diagnosis.[5] One practitioner claimed that among the group of 143 irises, he had correctly diagnosed 88 per cent of the patients with kidney disease. By itself, this is a very impressive statistic—he missed only 12 per cent of the cases of kidney disease. However, in looking at this practitioner's other results, it was shown that he had also diagnosed kidney disease in 88 per cent of the healthy volunteers. In other words, his discriminating ability between healthy and sick people was close to zero.

Iridology illustrates one of the characteristics of the thinking of alternative healers as they try to understand how the body works. To the conventional doctor, the eye has a very specific function and all its components are dedicated to achieving that function in the best possible way. The lens focuses light to produce the sharpest possible image on the retina. The cells of the retina interact to detect very small amounts of light. The iris, the coloured ring around the dark hole of the pupil, acts like the variable aperture in a camera opening and closing to adjust to the amount of ambient light. So in conventional medicine, an analysis of the eye will focus very specifically on the job of vision.

For the iridologist, however, the eye has another function. The eye is not only the organ of sight but a mirror of the health of the entire body. Iridologicial texts carry detailed diagrams categorizing different radiating segments of the iris as linked to, or providing information about, different organs and systems in the body. The skeleton, for example, is represented with the skull area at about two o'clock in the right iris and ten o'clock in the left; each set of leg bones stretches from the pupil down to six o'clock; and the other bones are arranged around the rest of the iris. Some iridologists even believe that if you snip a small piece of the iris out during an eye operation, it will have an effect on the organ corresponding to that piece. Some of the theory is backed up by an anatomical explanation; iridologists believe that there are 28,000 nerve fibres in the iris, far more than would be necessary to help it expand and shrink the pupil, and that these nerve fibres carry messages from all parts of the body and induce changes in the radiating bands of pigmentation in the iris as and when the parts of the body themselves change in some way, usually by acquiring some disease or abnormality.

What the iridologists believe about the eye is not generally accepted by conventional doctors, because they can find no evidence or proof for the iridological view. The iridologists, on the other hand, believe that any success they may have in making diagnoses proves the validity of their philosophy. This difference—between the conventional and the complementary views of the same organ— is typical of many of the differences between the two schools of medicine that we shall encounter later in this book. It also illustrates the difficulty in deciding the appropriate form of proof or evidence. Conventional doctors would require proof that iridologists can make accurate diagnoses and that those diagnoses are proven by other tests (such as X-rays or biopsies). Iridologists, on the other hand, would not require such stringent proofs of their techniques if the patients get better after using natural remedies for the problems they have diagnosed. Iridology, therefore, offers a neat example of the way in which two schools can both claim victory for their methods—but are both playing by different rules. It is only when careful and detailed studies (such as the one mentioned above) are carried out that a measure of true reproducibility can be obtained.

THE TREATMENT

If diagnosis seems complex and multi-factorial, treatment is infinitely more so.

Janice Martin, the legal secretary with the back injury, spends an hour under the healer's hands. For most of the time, the healer breathes heavily and makes comments about the energy fields around Janice. She touches Janice occasionally during the therapy. At the end of the session, Janice gets up from the couch with far greater ease than when she first lay down on it. She stands up and says that she is completely pain-free—for the first time in two and a half years.

In Sante Fe, a woman stands in front of a cabinet containing several hundred crystals and rocks. Under the eye of the crystal-therapist, she selects the ones that she likes best ("the ones that speak to you") and arranges them in a pattern on the carpet. The crystal therapist explains the significance of the stones and of the pattern. Then after the woman lies down, she lays the crystals on top of her body and adds a few others from the cabinet. She talks the patient through a process in which she has to imagine herself moving out through her emotional body, through her mental body and to the outer limit, her spiritual body. Then she reverses the process and the session ends.

Darren, the 12-year-old with appendicitis, is taken to the operating room where a small incision is made in the right iliac fossa. His appendix is found to be tucked behind the part of the bowel called the caecum, and when it is freed it looks red and inflamed. It is removed and sent to the pathology laboratory, which confirms that he had true appendicitis. Darren recovers perfectly from the operation and leaves hospital seven days later with his appendix in a bottle to show his friends.

Bill McConnell is the man of 58 with angina. Having had the coronary angiogram, the next day he goes back to the same room where another slender catheter is pushed, via the femoral artery, into his partly blocked coronary artery. This catheter has a little balloon at the end which is slowly and carefully inflated, cracking the plug of cholesterol-laden deposit that is blocking the artery. The remnant of the blockage will be absorbed by the body. A few months later, a follow-up angiogram shows that the artery is clear. Bill never suffers another attack of angina.

In New Mexico, Dale, the Navajo man with melancholia, watches while the medicine man spends 40 minutes constructing an intricate and beautiful painting made entirely of different-coloured sands on the floor of the *hogan* (hut). When it is complete, Dale and the medicine man participate in a ceremony in which corn pollen is scattered onto the sand painting. After that, the medicine man carefully destroys the sand painting and gathers up the debris to take it out to a special spot on the hillside (facing east) where he disposes of the sand with a further blessing.

Each of these events represents an intervention in our lives that is designed to correct the problem—the healing act. This can vary from the most visible (e.g., open-heart surgery) to the totally invisible (aura healing). Substances (homeopathic remedies, coffee enemas) may be given by the healer to the patient or the transaction may be apparently intangible but still assumed (by both parties) to be real (e.g., throwing of the chi, spiritual healing). It may take a moment (as with the American healers called *traiteurs*) or it may take years (psychoanalysis). It may have no side effects whatsoever or its side effects may be so severe that they threaten even the life of the patient (chemotherapy).

Treatment is what people really go to healers for. There are few patients who will be completely satisfied if their healer simply tells them what's wrong with them and does nothing about it. The purpose of the visit is clearly to get something done about the problem, and diagnosis is only the first step for most of us. In fact, we are positively disgruntled if we are told, "You have got coryza and there is nothing I can do about it," whereas if we were told, "I don't know what's the matter with you but this pill will certainly cure it," we might be puzzled but we would certainly feel that nine-tenths of our objective had been achieved.

An ill person—like nature—abhors a vacuum.

THE STAGE AFTER TREATMENT

It is sometimes said by physicians in private practice (in their rare moments of frivolity) that once a treatment has been given by a doctor to the patient, both parties await the next stage with a mixture of hope, anticipation and anxiety—the next stage being the doctor's presentation of the bill for his services.

Some form of payment or reward is an inevitable side effect of the consultation. (In Victorian times, it was generally felt that there were two inevitable outcomes—the doctor's bill and the death of the patient.[6]) However, the size or magnitude of that reward and the method by which the healer receives it vary considerably.

In London, a surgeon who is rich and famous as a result of his discreet dealings with the rich and famous gets approximately £1500 for a hernia repair operation that takes about half an hour. In Toronto, a medical oncologist gets $120 for an initial consultation lasting about an hour and a quarter. In a small *hogan* in the Navajo nation, New Mexico, a medicine man after conducting a blessing ceremony (including an intricate sand painting) receives a small blue cornmeal loaf that has been baked in the ground and some corn pollen (unless the blessing required something to do with the patient's defence, in which case he'll get an arrowhead). In a bayou near New Orleans, a *traiteur* will be rewarded with whatever the patient can afford. It'll probably be about $10. In Santa Fe, New Mexico, a top-notch crystal-therapist gets $400 for a two-hour session.

Not only are the payments varied, but the method by which the healer receives the reward also differs from place to place. The most popular method world-wide is direct reward—the patient pays the healer. Sometimes this is based on success (as used to be the practice in most of Europe—healers' bills tended to be ignored if the outcome wasn't satisfactory). In some places, the government acts as paymaster (for example, in Britain, Canada and Sweden) by means of health insurance. While healthy, every citizen contributes to the insurance fund from which he or she collects when the need arises. The healthy support the sick. In the United States, health insurance is much more complex and of the 260 million inhabitants, approximately 40 million have no health insurance at all. In other parts of the world, perhaps fittingly, healers are rewarded for keeping their patients healthy and are paid accordingly; if too many patients fall ill, the healer's income goes down. It is interesting to speculate what would happen if this method were introduced into medicine in the United States.

It's also interesting to note how the different countries decide to share their wealth among their healers—or rather, doctors. Britain spends 5.6 per cent of its gross national product (GNP) on health, Canada spends 8.5 per cent and the United States spends 11.3 per cent. Despite the hopes of the rich, wealth and health are not inextricably linked to each other.

Some conclusions may be drawn from these examples. First, different societies hold their healers in different degrees of awe, admiration and respect. Some cultures elevate their healers to the level of a quasi-priesthood, if not minor deities. Other societies respect their healers as important participants—pillars of the community—whose word is to be trusted and who play an important role in the general and non-medical life of their surroundings as well as in the health of the community. Others regard the healer as a tradesman who may or may not succeed at his or her job.

In every case, however, there is a statement being made—what occurs between the patient and the healer is, in some respects, a transaction and that transaction has a value. The precise value of the transaction is determined by society, by the market forces at work in that society and, of course, by the patient's ability to pay (or sue instead).

THE OUTCOME

Once the treatment has been given and a suitable time period has elapsed (suitable as determined by the nature of the disease, the treatment and the healer's knowledge of both) there are only three things that can happen. The patient's problems may get better, they may get worse or they may stay the same. Whether the problems are symptoms (such as pain, nausea or weakness), signs (such as bruising or jaundice) or investigations (such as anaemia or high blood pressure), there are still only these three possible outcomes.

Since much of the rest of this book (chapters five to eight) are centred for the most part on the outcome of therapy, we shall not deal with outcome measurements and analyses in detail at this point. However, it is worth remembering that whether the therapy costs a million dollars or a single cowrie shell, and whether the healer's analysis is a 50-page report or a single curt nod, there are still only three possible outcomes. The patient's problems may get better, they may get worse or they may stay the same.

THE START OF THE RELATIONSHIP

We have seen that the first meeting of a patient with a healer has certain unvarying and essential components, however different the encounters may appear at first sight. We have also established that the first consultation contains many aspects that are subjective and are determined, not by external biological factors, but by the attitudes of the individual patient and the individual healer—attitudes that are themselves partly determined by the prevailing culture and society.

Having established the common factors in the healer-patient consultation, we can now use the same process to look at the common factors in the treatment that the healer administers to the patient.

4. A TAXONOMY OF HEALING

In those situations where an alternative therapy works, the fact that we don't know why it works should, perhaps, be no more shocking than the same ignorance that still applies in many conventional medical treatments, particularly pharmacology.

TREATMENT

As we've seen, most patients seek out healers because they want to be treated. There are relatively few consultations in which a patient has no expectations of receiving one form of treatment or another. Even a visit for the sole purpose of being reassured that you *haven't* got the condition you feared involves "treatment" of that anxiety with reassurance.

At first glance, there seem to be hundreds of different kinds of treatment available, and they seem to vary in every aspect: in type, potency, side effects, duration, expense, patient participation, and location. Yet all of them—in both conventional and alternative medicine—can be subdivided into categories based on the fundamental type of action that the healer takes to assist the patient. Despite the fact that treatments seem to come in such a wide and bewildering variety of guises and appearances, there are actually very few basic ways in which a doctor or a healer can intervene to help a patient. In fact, it is possible to divide them into as few as five categories.

Our purpose in classifying methods of treatment in this way is not to suggest that this is the only possible way of considering treatments, but to show that there are superficial resemblances between treatments that arise from radically different philosophies of human biology and disease. This is not a matter of one form of therapy imitating another. Complementary practitioners sometimes appear to be imitating the actions of conventional doctors. Behaving this way may seem like an attempt to earn more respect or status, but, in fact, it is more usually a response to the constraints of human biology. There is a limited number of ways to influence the course of an illness. As we shall see, this means that a treatment cannot be easily assessed simply by looking at its form and outward appearance. So here's a simple taxonomy of healing methods:

Ingestive: in which the patient swallows a substance (or inhales it or receives it by enema).

Invasive: in which the healer's treatment involves the breach of the skin or mucous membranes of the patient.

External: in which the healer moves or manipulates some part of the patient's body without invading the skin, or else applies a substance (such as a poultice or plaster) to it.

Remote: in which the healer does not make direct contact with the patient's body.

Mental: in which the source of the healing is inside the patient's mind, and the role of the healer is to place that power within the patient's control.

INGESTIVE

In conventional medicine, most patients visiting their family practitioners assume they will be given a prescription of some sort. They expect to take it away and have it turned into a drug for self-administration, which they may (or may not) take according to the doctor's recommendations. This is ingestive therapy and it is so everyday and commonplace that we do not question it for a moment. Yet behind even the simplest prescriptions, there is a long history of observation, ingenuity and research.

Hilary Thompson is a 42-year-old woman who has come to her family practitioner with a history of trouble when she passes urine. For the last day and a half, she has had burning when she passes urine, has had to pass urine every two hours and has noticed a slightly rusty or smoky colour to the urine. She thinks that there is a smell associated with it. Her family practitioner examines her and finds nothing wrong. He takes a sample of the urine and writes out a prescription for one of the two commonest antibiotics used in urinary infections. Hilary starts taking the tablets and within 12 hours the symptoms have improved. In 24 hours they have disappeared.

This story is so common, one might think there is nothing to say about it. Yet that visit—and the prescription resulting from it—is based on a large amount of accumulated data and experimentation.

Infections of the bladder have been known since Hippocrates' time. In previous centuries they were the most frequent cause of stones in the bladder, a condition so common that there was an entire specialty of surgeons who did nothing except "cut for stone" to remove them. With the discovery of microbes, it was realized that infections of the bladder were usually caused by bacteria, most often of the same kind that came from the lower bowel. With the discovery of antibiotics that can kill these particular kinds of bacteria, bladder infection suddenly became a curable minor illness, instead of a recurrent or chronic misery. In Hilary Thompson's case, the urine sample was sent to the microbiology lab where it was plated out onto a culture medium, and in a day or so bacterial colonies were seen that were shown to be *Escherichia coli*. These colonies were simultaneously tested with little paper discs impregnated with antibiotics, and in Hilary's case the best antibiotic is a combination of a sulphonamide (sulphamethoxazole) and an antimalarial drug (trimethoprim), which work better together than when used singly. This is lucky, because Hilary's family doctor, suspecting that this would be the case anyway and knowing that Hilary is not allergic to sulpha drugs, had started her on precisely that combination even before the test results were known.

As with conventional medicine, ingestive methods of giving remedies are very popular among complementary practitioners. One of the more formal and highly institutionalized systems of prescribing is that of homeopathy, which provides a telling example of how different philosophies and different belief systems may produce results that are superficially very similar.

> Ellen Pascoe is 70. She is visiting a homeopath because she finds it difficult to cope with life. Thirty-four years ago, she had an operation for prolapse of the womb, during which the surgeon accidentally cut into one of her ureters (tubes that lead urine from the kidney to the bladder). This required a further operation to relocate the ureter. Ellen feels that the alteration to her system has made some difference to her.[1] She also has to take potassium tablets for her blood pressure. After the initial long consultation, which involved lengthy descriptions of all Ellen's major emotional traits and personality characteristics, her homeopath has prescribed a remedy derived from sepia, the ink of the cuttlefish. This has been chosen because in the homeopathic pharmacopoeia, sepia has a "symptom picture" of tiredness, weakness and a dragging-down sensation, often accompanied by an actual prolapse of the womb. The sepia remedy is also recommended for someone who has a desire for vinegar, pickles and tasty foods and a dislike for fat, meat and milk. These features apparently described Ellen very accurately when she visited the homeopath. Shortly after starting to take the sepia tablets, Ellen begins to feel better and is also able to stop taking the potassium tablets.[2]

Homeopaths believe that all diseases create some kind of imbalance in the harmony of the body and that the symptoms are not a direct result of the disease process itself but are an indication of the body's attempts to redress the upset balance. This is comparable to the fact that a fever is part of the body's defence against an infection. But whereas in conventional treatment, the physician would prefer to treat the infection (if possible) rather than simply bring the temperature down, the homeopath treats the symptoms. One implication of this approach is that one patient may need different treatment from another with the same disease. This is a direct result of the principle that "like cures like," and if a patient presents with a particular symptom or symptoms, the correct homeopathic remedy to prescribe is one which would *cause* those symptoms in a healthy person. Clearly, then, it is not enough to define an illness in the conventional medical way, in terms of infective organisms, autoimmune reactions or inborn errors, since each patient's body may respond to the initiator of the disease in a different way and require a different treatment. There is an important place for the patient's mental and emotional aspects, as well, in deciding what to prescribe. The patient is asked questions that seek to discover whether he or she has experienced any recent bereavement, fright, anxiety or deep-seated smouldering resentment, whether he or she prefers certain positions for sleeping, sweats unduly, avoids or seeks particular types of food, and so on. The symptoms the homeopath is interested in are often a long way from the things that drive patients to a conventional doctor. In an ongoing course of therapy, the patient is expected to record his symptoms as a guide to his progress to present to the homeopath. One of the thousands of such symptoms the patient is expected to record is: "After dinner, disposition to sleep; the patient winks." Such observations, combined with the answers to his questions and many more, lead the homeopath to choose a particular homeopathic remedy or several of them that are known or believed to cause the particular complex of signs and symptoms reported by or extracted from the patient.

In this whole process there are similarities and differences in comparison with conventional medicine. The investigation is thorough and systematic, and having arrived at a diagnosis, the homeopath turns to some data base that he has been taught to use—a collection of descriptions of drugs and the symptoms they are best used to treat. In the case of conventional medicine, these data about treatment have been obtained by cautious experimentation with patients; with homeopathy, too, there has been a systematic attempt to assess which remedies are appropriate for particular patients. The keystone of homeopathic therapy, however, is fundamentally different from drug testing in one important aspect. A conventional medical research project will move from a scientific theory about a drug to some form of practical test, initially in animals and then in humans. If these steps are successful, the experimenter will be justified in recommending the treatment to others to use, and it will eventually get into the textbooks. In homeopathy, the tests that are done to determine what to use with a patient, called "provings," are carried out in a different way. Here, various doses of a range of substances, usually derived from plants or minerals, have been administered over a long period to healthy volunteers. These volunteers have noted down what effects these doses have produced in their bodies—any symptoms or signs, changes in attitude or emotions, psychological problems and so on. Those changes that occur most commonly with the volunteers are then defined as the symptoms which that particular remedy should be used to treat.

So, to quote one example, as a result of provings, a dilute solution of potassium bichromate is recommended for patients with the following indications: thick, stringy, gelatinous or ropy green or yellow discharges from the mucous membranes of the eyes, ears, nose or throat; symptoms come and go suddenly and pains wander from place to place; joint pains often alternate with diarrhoea, respiratory problems or digestive upsets; patient gets cold easily and is worse in warm or hot weather; cough is often worse at 2 or 3 a.m. Presumably, if you give this substance to a healthy person it will *cause* some or all of this varied list of complaints.

Here, then, in homeopathy and antibiotic prescribing are two seemingly straightforward examples of ingestive therapy. The patient goes to the healer with a set of symptoms. The healer writes out a prescription (or makes up a mixture) based on his or her understanding of those symptoms, and the patient swallows it.

The choice of substance is based on the healer's understanding of the patient's symptoms, of the mechanisms by which diseases arise, of the way in which treatments work and on the healer's knowledge of specific treatments and experience in matching the treatment to the individual patient's situation.

In other words, the apparently simple act of reaching for a prescription pad or a bottle of medicine is a complex action rooted in the philosophy of the type of healing practised by that particular healer. Thus the philosophy of each particular type of healing is not an intellectual afterthought, like a piece of icing spread over the cake to make it look good after baking. The philosophy of each school of healing is fundamental to every act of its healers. As we shall see in later chapters, it is this that makes the most significant differences between the various disciplines, despite any superficial resemblances between their *modi operandi*.

INVASIVE

Invasive procedures are always more dramatic (and often more painful) than ingestive therapies. In the act of breaching the patient's skin or mucous membranes, the healer is making an irrevocable decision. There can be no doubt of the occurrence of an invasive action— the healer either does it or he (or she) does not. Whatever the procedure, the decision whether to carry it out (and how to do it) is an important one.

In conventional medicine, invasive methods of treatment are very common, are often high-profile and highly thought of by most patients. They are also highly rewarded, in that under most health services, a healer who cuts something is paid more than a healer who just writes something or talks. We've already seen two conventional examples of invasive healing—Darren's appendix was removed and Bill McConnell's coronary artery was unblocked with an inflatable balloon at the tip of a catheter.

Complementary medicine also has one or two invasive methods of healing.

In Ealing, West London, Anne Dawson, a 58-year-old woman, goes to seek the advice of Mr. Ho because she has bad headaches. The headaches come on approximately once a week, usually towards the end of the week, and are usually more severe if she has been under stress. There has been a lot of stress lately. She is separated (on a not very friendly basis) from her husband. Her youngest daughter lives with her, and there are constant arguments at home. There are many financial problems, and she has a long-running dispute with her landlord. She smokes and feels that she is at least 15 pounds over her ideal weight.

Today, Mr. Ho tells her, she will require treatment with 12 acupuncture needles. He uses alcohol swabs to clean small areas of skin on her hands, arms, scalp and ear lobes. He rapidly inserts small acupuncture needles into the skin so that the points are just submerged in it. He does not use the ancient technique of twirling the needles, but instead connects each of them to a small box that generates electric currents. According to acupuncturists, this has exactly the same effects as twirling the needles. He leaves the patient connected to the box for 20 minutes, then disconnects the needles and removes them from her skin. After 12 sessions of acupuncture, Mrs. Dawson's headaches are fewer and briefer, her cigarette consumption is reduced and she says that her energy level and mood have both improved noticeably.

As with ingestive medicines, there are certain resemblances between the invasive therapy used in the cases of Bill McConnell and Anne Dawson. Each of the treatments is based on the accumulated wisdom of many generations of practitioners.

Just to illustrate the background, let's look at the angioplasty done on Bill McConnell. The procedure depends on the knowledge that the chest pain we call angina is caused by disease in the arteries inside the heart (a fact known to the ancient Romans). However, direct demonstration of that disease was not even remotely feasible until the 1930s, when a brave young physician, Werner Forssmann, put a catheter into his own heart to prove that it could be done and so started the modern era of angiography. The device used to treat the artery, the balloon catheter, was invented originally for use in blocked arteries of the legs and only within the last ten years or so has it come into widespread practice for coronary arteries. Much research has now been published in which this procedure, called balloon angioplasty, has been used in different groups of patients with heart disease, looking for those that did best after the procedure. (It was such studies that showed angioplasty was useful in patients who, like Bill McConnell, have a single vessel blocked to more than 60 per cent of its diameter.)

Exactly the same sort of process has gone on with acupuncture, except that, as far as we can tell, it occurred many centuries ago. We assume that the current maps of the meridian points include only those points that have proved to be useful in practice over the millenia. A needle in the web of the thumb has been found to improve gallbladder pain, a needle behind the ear is known to produce improvement with respiratory difficulties, and so on.

Yet again, then, there are resemblances between the treatments. But as with ingestive remedies—and all therapies, for that matter— what the healers do is firmly bound up in the way the healers think, the way they view disease and the way they imagine the treatment works. The cardiologist sees angina as a pain caused by the accumulation of atheroma in the coronaries, which in turn is caused partly by inherited tendencies and partly by life-style habits such as smoking and lack of exercise. The acupuncturist sees angina as an imbalance of the chi, the energy field that flows through the body. Imbalances of the chi can best be remedied by direct interference with the flow of chi, which requires the insertion of needles into the mainline paths of the energy flow.

So it seems that many treatments depend not merely on the philosophy of the particular school of healing, but also on its store of accumulated wisdom and experience.

EXTERNAL

External therapy could be defined as either the application of substances (including plasters, poultices, liniments, unguents, aromawraps and many others) to the exterior of the patient's body, or else manipulation of the body without invading the skin. Both practices are extremely ancient traditions that probably precede recorded history. Both have interesting histories, but for the moment we shall focus on manipulation.

At various points in the past, manipulation has been viewed as something apart from mainstream medicine. In mediaeval Europe, there were practising bonesetters who were known for their skill in setting fractures. Although their modern descendants, orthopaedic surgeons, are highly respectable members of the medical fraternity, the mediaeval bonesetters were regarded as a sub-species of middle-grade manual labourer, quite distinct from the contemporary physicians who almost certainly brought much less relief to their patients.

The modern-day descendant of mediaeval manipulation in conventional medicine is physiotherapy.

John Roberts has a long-standing arthritis that has left him with widespread wasting of many muscles and chronic inflammation of several joints. Although the condition is now relatively quiescent, he has been left with frozen shoulders (meaning that he cannot lift his arms much above his head or turn them to scratch his back). The shoulder muscles are also markedly wasted and scarred, which has reduced the mobility of the arms yet further.

Twice a week he goes to the physiotherapy department where his physiotherapist, Diana, asks him to lie on his back. She takes one arm and brings it backwards over his head. She does another four different manipulations with that arm and then repeats the exercises with the other. After that, John does some exercises with pulleys and weights and then Diana wheels in a curious and old-fashioned-looking machine, although it is actually modern (made in 1988). It administers electric currents through a variety of blue and red sucker cups that are applied in pairs to the skin on both shoulders. Each cup holds an electrode, which is thus pressed tightly onto the skin. Diana turns up the current until John begins to feel uncomfortable and the muscles around his shoulder begin to twitch. She then turns down the current slightly and leaves him for 15 minutes. At the end of the procedure, he gets dressed and leaves with his shoulders still tingling slightly.

That's a fairly straightforward example of conventional manipulative therapy—and at first sight, the complementary equivalent doesn't look very different.

Padma is a woman with osteoarthritis affecting both hands and the right knee. Her chiropractor has X-rayed her entire body to confirm the misalignment of her skeleton and now does a long and complex series of bendings and stretchings of Padma's limbs and back. In particular, he concentrates on her neck and uses a spring-loaded device that administers swift (and almost painless) thumps to various parts of her body. After about 40 minutes of manipulations and exercises, the chiropractor repeats his initial assessment of Padma's legs and demonstrates to their mutual satisfaction that the misalignment has been partially corrected. So far, Padma feels only slightly better. But she'll be back for more next week.

In the previous two categories of therapy—ingestive and invasive—we have seen that the philosophy of the healer influences the therapeutic decision that he or she makes. Within the field of osteopathy, however, there are two quite distinct schools of philosophy. The limited or pragmatic school of osteopaths believes that its system of manipulation of the back (and attached limbs) is the best method of improving back pain and some joint pains. The older "classical" school of osteopathy believes that *all* diseases manifest themselves by an imbalance in the spine and that correct manipulation of the appropriate part of the spine will improve the disease, no matter where in the body that disease might be. Quite clearly, these two schools of thought make entirely different claims for the benefits of osteopathy and at present adherents to the limited school outnumber the classical school.

Practitioners from each of these schools of osteopathy might perform the same manipulations of the spine, but for entirely different reasons. So here is a case where the underlying thinking within a field of healing does not affect the form of treatment itself, but does affect what the healer hopes to achieve with it.

As for physiotherapy, this is one area of conventional medicine that is based, almost exclusively, on empiricism. The tradition of physiotherapy is a long one, and it is practised by trained therapists who are not doctors but who have a knowledge of anatomy, rheumatology, orthopaedics, respiratory medicine and so on, as well as the different techniques and manoeuvres that are their stock in trade. They practise as clinically independent personnel under the auspices of the Department of Physical Medicine (or Rehabilitation or Rheumatology and Rehabilitation, depending on the hospital) and are supervised by—and are the responsibility of—the doctor who is the head of that department. Many of the procedures that they use have been tested in trials and their benefit has been proven, but a larger number are simply techniques that have been used in practice for generations and that seem to produce benefit in many cases.

One may conclude from this pair of examples that even a manoeuvre as apparently simple as manipulation may have different schools of thought underlying it, and even when the manipulation is identical (as in the two groups of osteopaths) the motive and the philosophy behind them may be different.

The three categories of healing so far—ingestive, invasive and external—have seemed, at the very least, to be highly practical and highly physical. In the next two categories, there may be no physical elements at all.

REMOTE

In remote healing, there is no direct contact between the patient and the healer. In both conventional and complementary remote healing, the source of the healing power is external to both the patient and the healer. Usually it is invisible and has no physical manifestations of its presence apart from the effect on the patient.

In the radiotherapy department of a cancer centre in Toronto, Mrs. Davenport, a woman of 54, shows up for her first radiotherapy treatment. She has already had a planning appointment during which X-rays of her left breast were taken and measurements were made. These were based on the area of the breast from which a cancer had been removed by the surgeon, who had placed small metal clips at the borders of the operation so that an X-ray would reveal where the tumour had been.

The pathology report showed that there was a small clump of cancer cells (a fraction of a millimetre across) very close to the margin of the removed tumour, and the radiotherapist has decided to give the customary dose of radiotherapy to the breast, plus an extra "boost" dose to the place where the tumour was. The radiotherapist knows from her reading of the world literature that the boost will reduce the chance of a local recurrence of the cancer just as if the cancer had not reached the edge of the excised area.

Mrs. Davenport's breast and chest wall is covered in ink marks and lines. The radiotherapy machine looks like a space cannon from a 1950s sci-fi movie and is moved into the correct position by various motors controlled by the technologist. The technologist leaves the radiotherapy room, and the patient is alone. The door is closed and the radiotherapy machine is activated for a minute or so. There is no sound or smell and Mrs. Davenport feels nothing. The full course of therapy will require a daily treatment like this, five days a week for about five weeks. At the end of it, the skin over the breast is temporarily reddened for a few weeks and slightly darkened as if sun-tanned for a few months, but the contour and the shape of the breast will hardly have altered. Filling in a questionnaire on her opinion of the treatment one year after therapy, Mrs. Davenport states that she is "extremely pleased" with the final result.

Now consider another example of remote healing, this time from the realm of complementary medicine.

Wayne Morrison is a 65-year-old retired surgeon from Washington, D.C. He has enjoyed relatively good health since retiring, but has some difficulty with his bowels. In fact, intermittently he has quite severe constipation which, on a couple of occasions, has required enemas to relieve. Over the last few years, he has become involved with some remote healers in Santa Fe. They initially analyzed his blood (on a filter paper) and have been treating him at a distance by concentrating on his medical problems and transmitting healing waves into his etheric field. So far, it seems to have worked very well.

Today he telephones to say that he is constipated once again. The healers take a full history from him and then tell him what they are going to do and which of their remedies (which he already has at his home) he should take. At the appropriate time, the healers sit down and concentrate on Dr. Morrison and his bowel problems. They call on spiritual forces working at the level of the etheric field to alter the vibrations within Dr. Morrison's body and fix his constipation. The next day, Dr. Morrison telephones to tell them that, yet again, the treatment has worked. His bowels have opened. He is a happy man and his cheque is in the mail.

In remote healing, faith is crucial and central to the interaction between the patient and the healer. At first glance, perhaps radiotherapy is similarly an act of faith. After all, neither the patient nor the doctor can see the radiotherapy beam. Both of them can see the machine and the control dials, but neither of them can know that the amount of radiotherapy that is supposed to come out of the machine in fact does so. It is worth spending a moment considering the differences in the two uses of the word "faith" here, since this casts light on the nature of scientific proof in general and demonstrates that not all statements such as "I believe it" mean the same thing. Again, we need to stress that we are involved in value judgements on this issue. Differences in the basis of belief do not undermine the value of that belief to the patient (or the healer); we are simply examining the different foundations on which various beliefs may rest.

Radiotherapy is a high-dose version of the X-rays that are used in diagnosis. In fact, X-rays were discovered by the German scientist, Wilhelm Roentgen, in 1895 and his rays were first used to treat breast cancer in Paris just before the turn of the century. The patient in Toronto thus has 100 years of tradition behind her treatment; however, that still does not mean that the treatment is more than an act of faith. What constitutes the proof of the existence of radiotherapy as a physical phenomenon is the accumulated science of radiophysics. By using photographic film, Roentgen originally demonstrated that rays were coming out of a tube in which a metal target was bombarded by electricity from a cathode. The film was kept sealed in a packet but when developed showed dark spots where the X-rays had fallen on it. When Roentgen put lead on top of the film, the rays were blocked. The same principle was used with a fluorescent screen—the X-rays lit the screen up and when Roentgen put his hand in front of the rays, he saw the shadow of his hand on the screen. Both of those methods (technologically advanced but basically the same) are used today in diagnostic X-rays.

From 1895 to the present era, there has been a vast accumulation of studies on X-rays. The entire field of clinical radiation physics is devoted to working out the doses and the schedules of radiotherapy treatment. Devices called dosimeters are used to test every radiotherapy machine regularly to ensure that the dose intended to be given is the dose that is actually given. Although Mrs. Davenport doesn't know it, her radiotherapy machine has been checked at its regular time, and when the dials indicate that a dose of so many centiGrays (units that used to be called rads) have been given, the dials are correct. Over the past 40 years or so, a large amount of research on the dosage of radiotherapy has been published. We know that a dose of approximately 5000 centiGrays is the best total for the human breast, and that damage to normal skin and tissue is minimal when the doses are given five days a week over four to five weeks. Studies at the particular hospital in Toronto where Mrs. Davenport had her treatment showed that of 200 patients treated like this, 90 per cent found the final cosmetic result good or excellent.

Therefore, despite the fact that Mrs. Davenport sees and feels nothing during the therapy, her act of faith is backed up by a large amount of scientific evidence. There is of course the very slim possibility—conspiracy theories being very popular these days—that everybody has been lying, and that Roentgen never existed, the published reports are fabrications and the radiotherapy machine has nothing more than a sun-ray lamp inside it.

Given, then, that radiotherapy although invisible has physical existence, we can see that Mrs. Davenport's act of faith is founded on scientific data. That does not, of course, imply that Mrs. Davenport *has* to have radiotherapy for her tumour—she might, for instance, have preferred to have the entire breast removed (and quite a few patients do prefer that to the bother of daily therapy). However, that decision would be a personal one, again based on facts (there are now many studies showing that radiotherapy after a lumpectomy for small tumours produces exactly the same end results as complete removal of the breast). In other words, Mrs. Davenport may accept that radiotherapy is what her doctor says it is because of the accumulated data, but still may or may not accept the treatment itself, depending on her own evaluation of the difficulty in going through five weeks of therapy compared to a larger operation.

When we look at spiritual healing, we see that at the moment of intervention, there is a similar act of faith on the part of the patient.

The patient cannot see or smell the force of the healing, although some patients feel a sensation of heat. The healer might state that the force of his healing comes from God through Jesus Christ (not all spiritual or charismatic healers are Christians and some do not belong to any church or institutionalized religion). This force is conducted to the patient via a special power given (unasked) to the healer. As in all matters of spirituality, there is no foundation of scientific data—by definition there cannot be. Spirituality by its nature involves faith. The fact that at present there are no data proving the existence of a spiritual healing force does not negate the belief itself. Although spiritual healing in this context is regarded as a branch of complementary medicine, there are other contexts in which spirituality is employed in medicine and is not regarded as complementary at all. This different context casts some light on the nature of what we label "alternative" or "complementary."

Ward C3 is a 36-bed ward in a large teaching hospital. It is the oncology ward for patients with cancer. Some are receiving therapy for their cancer (chemotherapy or radiotherapy) and some are being looked after when active therapy has become ineffective and the patient's condition is deteriorating. Mrs. Mason, a widow of 72, is a patient in the latter category. She has breast cancer that has spread to the bones and that has been held in remission for various periods of time over the last five years. Now the disease has become resistant to hormone therapy and chemotherapy. Mrs. Mason understands that there is no further effective therapy to try. She is physically free of pain (having had radiotherapy to her left hip, which previously hurt) but she is very troubled and distressed. Her two sons (in their late forties) have long-standing arguments and are both highly critical of each other, and quite often of their mother. Mrs. Mason has many regrets about her marriage (she was divorced before her husband's death) and about the way she spent her life. The doctor looking after her has had several long conversations during which she has poured out many of her troubles. He now suggests that the hospital chaplain visit her.

The chaplain sees Mrs. Mason for up to an hour on half a dozen occasions. They talk about God, about religion in general, about religious observances (Mrs. Mason feels guilty that she has not been a regular church-goer) and about the nature of spirituality. They pray together. After those sessions, Mrs. Mason tells her doctor that she feels much better and is far less troubled about her medical condition. She is noticeably more cheerful and is able to communicate more effectively and more closely with her sons.

Something occurred during the sessions between the chaplain and Mrs. Mason. She was referred to the chaplain by the doctor in the same way (and on the same type of referral form) that he would have requested physiotherapy for her. In Mrs. Mason's view, the doctor could not have done what the chaplain did, but he personally did not make the patient better; he only showed her the power of forgiveness and peace that came from God.

The example of Mrs. Mason is certainly not unusual (this was one of two dozen referrals to the chaplaincy that week). None of the staff would have regarded the visits as a form of alternative medicine, and nobody (Mrs. Mason included) expected the visits to affect the cancer or became disappointed when the medical situation was unchanged. The visits were set up in order to decrease her distress, and they achieved their objective.

Spiritual healing, although it resembles chaplaincy in many respects, has some important differences. Spiritual healers (as indicated by their title) believe that the process will achieve healing. Thus, there is a fundamental difference between chaplaincy and spiritual healing. In the latter it is expected that some healing will occur; in the former it is expected that spiritual distress will be relieved. The spiritual healers believe that there is a quite distinct force of healing that is channelled through them. Although it comes from God and Jesus—as does the sense of peace achieved in prayer—this is believed to be more than mere balm; it is a separate healing force of its own.

This "healing force" is not expected from the chaplain, but this does not diminish the perceived value of the chaplain's visits. No one in the hospital would say, "The chaplain is *only* relieving Mrs. Mason's spiritual distress." Relief of her distress is a thoroughly laudable aim in itself, and everyone concerned is impressed when it is achieved. The difference between chaplaincy and spiritual healing is based on the objectives and claims of the healer and therefore on the expectations of the patient.

To take this issue one step further, the co-existence of these two types of spiritual intervention raises some fundamental issues about mankind's attitude to religion and to magic. We shall be examining that in greater detail in the next chapter, but it is clear that there are major similarities between our attitudes to both of these belief systems. Religions in the Western world are generally systematized and have established social networks and patterns of observances and they can interrelate with the State (such as in school prayers, the national anthem and so on). Other belief systems, such as aura-healing, whether or not the individual healer requires the power of a deity, do not have widespread social recognition and are more individual systems that a patient can join voluntarily. One is regarded as the social norm, the others are not.

Clearly the role of religion and spirituality in healing is a major issue, and some areas of it are beyond the scope of this book. However, for the moment it may be permissible to consider spiritual healing and religious counselling as aspects of the same part of the human belief system. The major visible difference between them is that religions have widespread social acceptability—to the extent of being passed on involuntarily to children and recorded on secular forms—whereas spiritual belief systems are far less institutionalized and are more related to the individual directly.

However, both spiritual healing and chaplaincy are quite distinct from the final category of healing we will now consider—mental healing (both conventional and complementary), which does not require any external force, but which calls upon the mental reserves of the patient.

MENTAL

In Manchester, Mrs. Oldroyd, a woman of 45 with two teenage children, has been referred to a psychologist. She has had intermittent difficulties with her vision for just over a year. On three or four occasions, she has had double vision for several days at a time; on one occasion, she had pain behind her left eye that worsened when she looked to the side. She has also had some unsteadiness and clumsiness affecting sometimes the left leg and sometimes the right arm. Lately she has had some numbness and tingling around her mouth. She has been seen by a neurologist, who ordered a special test called Visual Evoked Potentials. He told her that her story, taken with the results of the test, confirmed the diagnosis of multiple sclerosis. Mrs. Oldroyd was devastated at the news. A flood of worries—about herself, her family, her finances, among others—threatened to overwhelm her. Over the subsequent days and weeks, she was perpetually anxious, was unable to sleep or eat properly and found herself close to tears much of the time. The neurologist thought she might benefit from the particular support services offered by the psychology department.

The psychologist spends half a dozen one-hour sessions with Mrs. Oldroyd. During these sessions, he listens to her story and her main problems. He encourages her to talk about and examine her attitudes to the illness and the future. Among other techniques, he uses a form of psychotherapy called cognitive therapy in which the patient is gradually helped to change her thinking about her situation. Over the course of the sessions, Mrs. Oldroyd is able to reduce the anxiety—and the distress—caused by the diagnosis. Neither Mrs. Oldroyd nor the psychologist believe that this therapy will affect the course of the multiple sclerosis, but both are pleased and impressed with the decrease in Mrs. Oldroyd's distress.

There is no mystery here. The psychologist has been trained in a conventional university and has learned the history and techniques of the major schools of psychotherapeutic thought. He has spent a year as an "intern" under the direct supervision of an experienced psychologist discussing every case (and his own reactions to every case) with him.

This particular psychologist is not upset or offended when he is called a healer. However, he would object to any suggestion that mysticism is involved in his technique. He believes that what he does is basically simple, although it requires experience and expertise in practice. He believes that part of the effect of his therapy is due to the considerable powers of concentration and understanding that he brings to the interactions. He feels that these are essential in order to focus accurately on the patient's problems and to help his patients use their own strengths and coping mechanisms to reduce pain and distress. The psychologist does not happen to believe in any external forces (he is an atheist) and does not believe that there are any forces at work in the interaction other than the action of one person's words on another's state of mind. He cannot explain precisely in every detail *how* he does what he does, but feels that the principles can be studied, analyzed and passed on to other trainees in the same way in which they were passed on to him.

Indeed, there are many studies of different types of psychotherapy, and cognitive therapy has been studied in several research centres. Its success rate is certainly less than 100 per cent and in the current state of knowledge, it is not known whether the failures are due to the wrong patients being selected for the therapy or the inexperience or inability of the therapist.

In an office in Tijuana, Mexico, Amy Francis, a young Californian woman who was diagnosed as having breast cancer six months previously, lies in a reclining chair. The man in the chair beside her is a physician, Dr. Tesselman, trained in psychiatry at a well-known American medical school. He is in private practice as a psychiatrist, specializing in visualization techniques and using them particularly with cancer patients. Ms. Francis closes her eyes, and Dr. Tesselman asks her to imagine herself relaxing near some water and to describe it. She selects a beach that she had happy memories of as a child and describes it. He asks for more details and adds ideas of relaxation and calm. When she is completely relaxed, Dr. Tesselman asks her to imagine her cancer and then to imagine the cells of her immune system. He asks her to visualize particularly the white cells and to see them as strong and vigorous. He asks her to see them as stronger than the weak cells of the cancer. He asks her to send messages of strength and success to the white cells.

The session lasts just under an hour. At the end of it, Ms. Francis slowly opens her eyes and sits up. She tells Dr. Tesselman that she feels much better and is not only more relaxed but more positive that her body is going to defeat her cancer.

In contrast to the psychotherapist, Dr. Tesselman does believe in a mysterious force. He believes that the change in attitude of Ms. Francis produces a change in the potency and behaviour of her immune system and will alter the course of the disease. However, like the psychotherapist, he cannot describe in detail precisely what he does, but he believes that fundamentally it is a simple process, although requiring some experience and expertise in practice.

Conclusion: The Same But Different?

In this brief survey of the different ways in which healers intervene to help their patients, we have seen that there are certain observable similarities between the techniques of conventional and complementary medicine. However, we have also seen that there are fundamental differences in the philosophies. At this point, then, the true differences between conventional and complementary treatments are not yet fully defined.

In fact, the superficial similarities between the treatments raise more questions than they solve. What are we to infer from the fact that auras and radiation are equally invisible to patients; that homeopathic pills and Librium look identical; that the reflexologist manipulating the foot looks as if he is doing something similar to the physiotherapist manipulating an elbow? Of course, one possible conclusion—and an insignificant one—that may be drawn from observing these similarities is that there is only a limited number of things you can do to a body, and that medicine (alternative or conventional) does most of them. But we believe there is a far more significant conclusion to be drawn if we look back at our comparative analysis in more detail. In our portraits of the various forms of therapy, we have tried to be as descriptive as possible. But we have also tried to give some indication of the *reasons* given by each practitioner for choosing one category of treatment, or modality, rather than another. And it is here that we begin to see a fundamental difference between the disciplines. If we ask a conventional doctor why he uses a drug rather than radiotherapy, or psychotherapy rather than surgery, he will answer in terms of a unified body of knowledge of anatomy, physiology, biochemistry and so on. These are separate but complementary ways of looking at the same thing. The *biochemistry* of the blood relates to a fluid that runs through the lungs and *physiologically* exchanges gases before plunging *anatomically* into the blood vessels and the heart. In choosing a method of treatment, the doctor tries to find the one that deals best with the illness—an illness that can be a malfunction of any of these biological characteristics. The doctor, usually a general practitioner, to whom the patient first presents his complaint, will therefore choose one of a number of colleagues to pass the patient on to if he can't treat him himself. *But whoever he sends the patient to will have exactly the same understanding of how the body works as the referring doctor.*

By contrast, look at the patient consulting the alternative practitioner. Of course, there is no such thing as a general practitioner of alternative medicine. For if there were, he or she would have to be able to believe several contradictory things at the same time. This healer would have to believe that his patient's problem could be a malfunction of his meridians, his zones, his chakras or his chi lines, and the healer would have to choose between these possibilities in order to send the patient to an iridologist, a radionics expert, a homeopath, a naturopath or an acupuncturist. Curiously enough, any alternative healer worth his salt will claim to be able to treat the vast majority of problems that cause patients to go to a healer. No acupuncturist ever said, "Your headache is one that is best treated by a homeopath"; no osteopath would say, "Your backache is just the kind that responds well to herbal remedies—let me send you to a herbalist." It seems to be the case that every alternative healer believes that his or her system provides a comprehensive account of how the body goes wrong and how it can be treated. Perhaps this is one of the most puzzling features of complementary medicine— the therapies all seem to have comprehensive and mutually exclusive explanations of the functions of the human body and of disease. How can all these apparently contradictory systems be correct at the same time?

For people practising and researching conventional medicine, this is a major objection to alternative therapies. They find little or nothing in any of the therapies that corresponds to what they have been taught about the body and how it works. The alternative therapist's description of how the body works is often phrased in terms of the whole person, with the physical body and its problems being only one part of a broader entity that is treated by the practitioner. Sometimes this need be no more than a minor difference of opinion. If healers wish to define psychological illness as being due to imbalances on the mental plane, while doctors call them neuroses or psychoses, the two descriptions may embody mere differences in language, and they can be seen as using different metaphors. But when a polarity therapist, say, diagnoses and prescribes on the basis of the existence of a series of "centres of energy" in the body—the etheric centre, the air centre, the water centre, the fire centre and the earth centre—and talks of energy flows and wireless circuits between those centres, we are getting beyond metaphor to a fundamental difference in understanding, and perhaps even in what are taken to be "facts." Almost every alternative therapy derives its course of action from a theoretical basis that is outside the conventional scientific understanding of how the body works and is sometimes in conflict with it. Even acupuncture meridians, part of a system that has shown some success in pain reduction, are undemonstrable in any meaningful physical sense, apart from those instances where they coincide with nerve pathways.

One complementary doctor uses a device that is designed to measure energy levels at acupuncture points all over the body, as a guide to the patient's health. When one patient was tested with the device, the doctor told him that it showed that the bits of him that were working least well were his pancreas and his liver or, in the doctor's words, "as the Chinese would call it, your spleen and your liver." When the patient was given two sophisticated liver function tests in a hospital shortly afterwards, they showed no abnormality at all. The doctor's explanation for the discrepancy reflected the way in which practitioners of forms of alternative therapy, who appear to be dealing with the same organs and systems of the body as conventional medicine, turn out to be dealing with very different concepts, even though they are using conventional words. "What the device is doing," said the doctor, "is looking at the liver in the *energetic* sense, as if you were doing a traditional Chinese diagnosis. The liver is the liver in conventional medicine but it's also the liver in traditional Chinese medicine, which is the same and slightly different."

A similar discrepancy arose when another of this doctor's diagnostic tests on the same patient, comparing his left side with his right, failed to show any imbalance, even though it turned out that the patient was partially paralyzed in his right arm and right leg, due to an inflammation of the spinal cord. Again, the doctor's explanation was counter-intuitive—"This test is not specifically designed to look at how your neurology is functioning. It is designed to look at how your acupuncture channels are functioning, and there is not necessarily a link between your neurological function or disfunction and your acupuncture channels' function and disfunction."

Such explanations make it very difficult to understand how, in any meaningful sense, the alternative therapies this doctor and his colleagues practise could address any of the conventional ills that people bring to their doctor, since at least one of his diagnostic techniques seems to find problems the patient is unaware of and miss problems that are only too present in his physical body.

Similar difficulties arise when trying to reconcile conventional science with the theoretical underpinnings of homeopathy. As we described earlier, the exact homeopathic prescription to use for a particular collections of symptoms was determined, some time ago in fact, by administering a succession of preparations to a group of healthy people and noting the effects. This process has proved to be very difficult to reproduce with other people given the same preparations. Furthermore, the preparations themselves, although derived from physical entities—molecules of plant chemicals or minerals—appear to behave like no other molecules. The remedies are considered to have the strange property of being more potent the more they are diluted. Most, if not all, homeopathic remedies have been diluted so much that they no longer contain any molecule of the original substance. One remedy, derived from the friable part of an oyster shell, is prescribed in a dose that consists of a hundredth of a millionth of a millionth of a millionth of a millionth of a millionth of a millionth of a millionth of a millionth of a millionth of a millionth of a grain of the shell. At this degree of dilution—and some remedies are prescribed at a greater dilution—there is no scientific test known to man that could distinguish between the "active" preparation and an identical pill without the homeopathic ingredient.

With each of the principle alternative therapies, its advocates attempt to justify the treatment with reference to an underlying rationale. In almost every case, the rationale is different from every other and, in general, it is difficult to relate any of them closely to the huge body of anatomical or physiological knowledge that has been built up by conventional medical and biological research over the last hundred years. And with some therapies, only a cursory attempt is made to offer any explanation at all.

None of the above can be taken as overwhelming objections to, or refutations of, the validity of alternative medicine. No conventional doctor would argue that we now know all we will ever know about how the body works. All good doctors are prepared for new knowledge and could even imagine a situation where new discoveries contradict old beliefs. And in those situations where an alternative therapy works, the fact that we don't know why it works should, perhaps, be no more shocking than the same ignorance that still applies in many conventional medical treatments, particularly pharmacology.

In the end, faced with a treatment that works, we must use it first and ask questions afterwards. Conventional medicine has always acted that way and alternative healers should be allowed the same licence. So, setting aside the question of scientific validity, we should look next at whether alternative healers succeed at their task. One indication of whether they do will emerge from an analysis in the next chapter of why people are visiting alternative practitioners in increasing numbers.

5. PHILOSOPHICAL ATTRACTIONS

Whatever the cause of the disease, the person who suffers from it is threatened with the loss of personal significance unless someone helps him or her rediscover it. Conventional doctors are rarely good at helping the patient with that process; complementary practitioners usually are.

In unprecedented and increasing numbers, patients are consulting practitioners of every type of alternative or complementary medicine. Between 1986 and 1992, the proportion of people in one sample who had used complementary medicine rose from one in seven to one in four. This shift is due partly to the attractions of complementary medicine and partly to dissatisfaction with conventional medicine. In this chapter we will look at the most common reasons for going to complementary practitioners and later at the main causes of dissatisfaction with conventional doctors. We shall therefore be excluding the millions of patients who are quite satisfied with their conventional doctors and also those patients (whose numbers are not known) who are dissatisfied with their complementary practitioners.

Patients are often attracted to one particular type of complementary medicine because it appeals to them as an entire package. So any attempt to divide and categorize the main sources of that appeal is bound to be somewhat artificial. Nevertheless, there seem to be two main categories: one is the philosophy inherent in complementary medicine's views of health and disease, and the other is a group of practical attributes that are associated with the healer and the remedy. In looking at these positive features of complementary medicine, we will also review the main sources of dissatisfaction with conventional doctors, particularly when they are compared to their complementary counterparts.

THE CONCEPT OF HEALTH

Most people probably think that doctors and hospitals have some effect on our health. After all, in the United Kingdom, the main body providing medical services is called the National *Health* Service, and most countries have a Ministry or Department of *Health* to control their own medical services. But in fact, of course, if you look at the way most conventional doctors spend their time, they are almost entirely preoccupied with *disease*.

And indeed, until fairly recently this was probably what people wanted most from their doctors—relief from the pain and distress that were a result of a whole range of diseases that were far more prevalent in society than they are today. But in recent times many people have come to think of *health* as a much more positive state, defined as something more than just the absence of disease. What's more, "being in a state of health" is seen as a basic human right, and whether or not it is the sort of right that can be enforced by legislation, it has certainly affected people's attitude to health care, to the extent that they look much more closely nowadays at how to become healthy as well as how to be free of disease. They also look to doctors, as traditional curers of disease, to help with that task.

While the aim of total health for all (or for all who want it) is, like motherhood, something that it would be very unpopular to argue against, it appears to be very difficult to achieve. Even at the level of disease elimination, medicine is trying to deal with a moving target. Diseases come and go; bacteria and viruses mutate; new aspects of the man-made world introduce new pathology; and even treatable diseases proliferate in societies that don't have the money or resources to treat them.

At the moment there are diseases (sometimes random, sometimes man-made) that deny the state of health to millions of patients. Furthermore, even in the absence of disease, it is doubtful whether the medical profession as currently trained and organized is the right organization to provide health.

The truth is that medicine has never been the major factor in improving the health of large populations; doctors are experts in changing the lives of seriously ill *individuals*, but are rarely as skilled in dealing with large communities. It has now been shown to the satisfaction even of doctors that the largest decreases in the most dangerous infections of this century occurred on a country-wide scale many years before the advances in medical science that brought about cures (or prevention) in individuals. Tuberculosis had already declined dramatically by the time streptomycin was introduced; scarlet fever and diphtheria had dwindled before vaccination; and polio was on the run long before the Salk and Sabin vaccines. This does not diminish the achievements of medical science—it is just that sanitation, housing and living standards in general have always been more important factors than medical advances in the true health of a population.

Until recently, this role of conventional doctors as treaters not preventers was not considered a problem by most people. Doctors were simply meant to be bringers of comfort and solace and expert diagnosticians who could tell the patient and family what was going to happen next, even when they were powerless to change it. It was accepted that doctors cured rarely and cared always.

Today, society's expectations have changed, and the medical profession is ill-equipped to satisfy those expectations. Even in those areas where doctors seem to be reaching beyond the curing of disease, such as screening for high blood pressure, cervical cancer, breast lumps, rectal cancer and so on, they are really detecting early disease rather than maintaining positive health.

Complementary practitioners almost always advertise health as the commodity in which they trade. Although some people who visit them have traditional medical complaints, others are not only free of disease by conventional definitions but are not ill by their own definitions. They do not feel ill but want to enhance their health. This motive for visiting a complementary practitioner contrasts sharply with patients' motives for seeing a conventional doctor. Very few people would consider going to a conventional doctor's office (apart from an annual check-up—more early detection) or a hospital outpatient department just to see if there was anything they could do to enhance their health. By contrast, complementary practitioners specialize in exactly this type of consultation. Some would have to consider another form of livelihood if it disappeared.

The concept of health as an objective seems to have become widely accepted without being examined critically or specifically defined. Many of the major causes of ill health are actually quite well known to scientists, doctors, epidemiologists and public health experts: they are associated with poverty, poor education, inadequate housing, drug and alcohol addiction and so on—so it is not difficult to envisage the eradication of these problems as a major source of improved health for large populations.

But most of the people who seek complementary medicine don't usually come from the social groups that suffer from these problems. The people who are most attracted to the idea of health are, on the whole, adequately provided for but who have expectations of achieving some higher state of existence that would be better characterized as "happiness" or "fulfilment" than health.

The definition is stretched yet further by some healers who equate health with personal *wealth* (and they mean *lots* of money, not merely the absence of poverty). Thus the subtext of health promotion has now gone beyond the prevention of preventable or treatable diseases (heart disease, cervical cancer and so on), beyond definitions of physical fitness and even psychological balance and is making the universal claim that "you could be happier—or richer—than you are now." Unlike most conventional medical claims, this hypothesis is almost impossible to refute. There are very few people who have sufficient self-confidence to say "No thanks, I'm as happy (or as rich) as I can possibly be." The adducement of more (of anything) rarely lets its promoters down, and health is no exception.

The idea that achieving total health is within the grasp of every individual may do some good by encouraging people to take more exercise and give up smoking, but it can have less beneficial side effects. In much of the complementary literature, it is strongly suggested that full health is not only within the power of everybody, but that it is also his or her *responsibility* to achieve maximum health. Although this may be true with specifically behaviour-related diseases (such as heart disease, lung cancer and obstructive airways disease associated with cigarette smoking), not every disease is within the realms of the individual's control, and it is not true to say that complete health is within everyone's grasp. In fact, while the "you can get it all" message is very positive and helpful for the healthy, it carries a stigma of blame and failure for the sick ("If I *could* have been healthy but I'm actually sick, it must be my fault").

This is not a mere philosophical quibble. Patients with serious illnesses—particularly cancer—are extremely vulnerable to feelings of guilt and rejection, and the constant reminder that they are in some way to blame for their poor state of health is both untrue and cruel.

The concept of health as the individual's responsibility is probably a major benefit of complementary medicine if you are healthy or if you are in the process of dealing successfully with a disease. If, on the other hand, the illness has not been caused by anything you have done, or if you are losing the battle against it, the same rallying cry can be damaging, demoralizing and punitive. Personal responsibility for health is a two-edged sword—one edge is a catchy slogan for the healthy, the other edge cruelly transforms the patient into a scapegoat.

ENERGIES AND FORCES

Many branches of complementary medicine embody the concept of a life energy or a vital force. Commonly this centres on the idea that a healthy state is the result of a correct balance of life forces and that diseases are the result of imbalances or a maldistribution of them. Even more crucial is the idea that life forces have an *inherent* tendency to balance themselves and that the patient can be healed or improved by enhancing nature's ability to rebalance the forces.

It is easy to see why this idea is appealing. First, it is relatively easy to understand compared with the incomprehensibility to most people of biochemistry, physiology and the other medical sciences, and it reinforces the widespread conviction that scientists don't know everything.

Most people outside the medical or scientific professions have only a dim memory of the scientific facts and concepts they learned at school, if indeed they learned anything at all. To them, therefore, all "new" ideas in this area start from the same base—ignorance—and can therefore seem equally plausible. What's more, with the help of a simple diagram and arrows that seem to link up in interesting ways, the explanation seems remarkably easy to understand. Patients experience as little scepticism towards the explanations of the acupuncturist or the homeopathist as they do towards those of the consultant endocrinologist. Both groups talk in terms of invisible, undemonstrable entities, and both groups wear a mantle of authority or at least have diplomas on the wall.

In fact, the overall concept of self-balancing life forces is not inherently implausible since there are analogous mechanisms at work in the human body. Most of the important chemicals in our blood are regulated within very strict limits. Oxygen, carbon dioxide, sugar, urea, potassium and sodium, for example, are all kept within the optimum range by our lungs, pancreas, kidneys and liver. However, that does not mean that every disease is subject to regulation by natural forces. In fact many diseases are linked to a "natural" *loss* of regulation. Diabetes, for example, is caused by a deficiency of insulin, and there is no force in the body that will substitute for it. If there is such a thing as the balance of life energy, it has let diabetics (and many others) down.

Concepts of life energy (involving pathways and fields called chi, auras, chakras and so on) do, however, seem to provide useful *metaphors* for people, and as such they should not cause anyone any major difficulties. It is when, like the concepts of health, they have been interpreted and exploited too widely and too literally—often with multiple layers of scientistic explanation—that the problems arise. "Life force" and "psychic energy" are too indefinable and too generalized to support claims that a specific intervention (whether it is shiatsu, reflexology, colour therapy or any other) must benefit a patient because it releases blocks in the flow of energy. As we shall see in later chapters, if any of these claims is literal, it should be examined critically. If a practitioner says, "I will intervene to help you use your life forces to heal you," it is quite legitimate and very important to ask, "How do you know the forces exist? Heal me of what? And can you prove it?" Which raises another appeal of complementary medicine: the idea of self-healing.

SELF-HEALING

Self-healing as used in alternative medicine refers to the capacity of the body, from within its own resources, to cure disorders that have in the past needed doctors and their remedies to treat. It is a concept bound up intimately with the ideas of health, life forces and nature. The word is used very widely to refer to those properties of the individual's body, mind or spirit that are capable of combatting disease or illness. Once again there is a lot of merit in the central idea. Healing is what happens when the body repairs a wound in the skin or a fracture of a bone: it implies restoration of the affected part to its previous state. When we get a cold, for example, the cold virus triggers a response that "educates" groups of white cells. Antibodies are produced that then alter the behaviour of other white cells and within a few days we kill the virus and our cold gets better. It would be quite legitimate to call this process "self-healing," though it would be more accurate to call it simply "healing," or, even better, "recovering." Problems arise when this idea is extended to explain the processes of chronic or severe diseases, and to suggest mechanisms of combatting them; for instance, many complementary schools subscribe to the idea that cancers develop because the natural healing processes of the body have failed or are blocked, and that many therapies—particularly mental or psychological ones—can unblock and release the self-healing powers and reverse the disease.

The first part of this belief—like the belief in life forces—has an equivalent in cancer biology; for example, in specimens of human cancers, one can isolate certain white cells (lymphocytes) that when grown in a dish (away from the cancer cells) are then capable of destroying other cancer cells and sometimes the cancer cells of the tumour in which they were found. Thus, in a very generous interpretation of the phrase "blocking the self-healing powers," the growing cancer is indeed somehow able to neutralize the abilities of these cells.

However, the direct application of this test-tube observation to the treatment of human patients with cancer is conjectural and probably unjustified. Sadly, there is a great gap between the neutralization of this specific defence mechanism at the cellular level and the idea that the body has any practicable self-healing powers against cancer that can be activated by that particular individual's mind or by any form of complementary medicine. (We shall look at this in greater detail in the next chapter.) But the idea is immensely attractive, it fits quite neatly into some of the newest work on hormones and neurology and if it were proven fact, one might be able to think of many different explanations by which such a phenomenon could be explained. Unfortunately, as we shall see, there is no evidence that it is true. Like life energies, self-healing is a useful metaphor for the human spirit, but, to date, it has not been shown to exist as an internal force capable of being harnessed by complementary practitioners to reverse serious diseases.

HOLISTIC

HEALER: I'd like you to look at my ring. Can you see all the facets that make a whole?

PATIENT: Yes.

HEALER: I believe that we do not use all the facets that are within us. And I see my job as being able to help you to take the veil away and use what you have within you. It's very exciting. It's very happy making. And I believe we only get better through great joy.

PATIENT: Yes.

HEALER: Also, it is a slightly different approach from medical science. Healing believes in holism. Which means you're not just body, are you? You react when you're not feeling well. So we are using the whole of you. And there is no reason why we cannot use your mind to help your body. Kindness to yourself. Kindness to the body. You'd do it for somebody else. Now you're going to do it for yourself. Now can you just tell me where you feel pain...

There are several meanings of the word "holistic" with which nobody could argue. The idea that a human being comprises at least three elements—mind, body and spirit—is perfectly reasonable since we can all define the word "spirit" in some way that includes aspects of emotions, feelings, conscience and motives, even if we do not believe in the existence of a separate soul.

In its most common use, holistic medicine can be defined as treating the entire patient and paying attention to disorders reflected in the mind, body and spirit, whatever their origin. Again, no sensible person could possibly argue with this, since it embodies the idea of dealing with the psychological and spiritual elements of illness. This applies to almost every scenario of illness imaginable. Even in the direst emergency—say an arterial haemorrhage—it is still worthwhile for the emergency surgeon to reassure the patient (if there is time) while preparing for surgery. And in the chronic diseases, to ignore the psychological and emotional repercussions of physical illness is to cause deep disaffection of the patient.

The holistic approach to the patient is therefore the central and most essential ingredient in all healing relationships, whether in conventional or complementary medicine. In fact, it was enshrined in the conventional doctors' Hippocratic Oath so that, in theory, all conventional doctors are supposed to have been treating every patient as a whole person at every visit. In practice, there has been a great deal of backsliding (particularly over the last four or five decades) and the true acknowledgement of the patient as a whole person became more theory and lip service than reality in much of conventional medicine.

The problems start when the definition of holism becomes overextended. The use of the word has now been stretched by practitioners of complementary medicine to include the idea that because the inter-relationship between mind, body and spirit is so close it must be true that the mind and spirit can change anything in the body. It is thus almost implicit within the idea of holism—and occasionally explicit in some complementary literature—that because mind, body and spirit are related, *any* disorders of the body, even potentially lethal ones, can be reversed by a change in mind or spirit. This extension of the holistic concept (like that of health as the individual's responsibility) has major implications for patients with serious diseases and should not be accepted as fact unless it can be clearly proven.

Proving that there are some links between mind, body and spirit is not enough in itself; for example, there is some fairly solid evidence that major psychological stress increases the likelihood of developing a cold in the nose after exposure to cold viruses. However, a cold is not a serious disease, and this observation in itself does not immediately imply that a change in attitude of mind or spirit will reverse serious diseases such as cancer. Improvements in state of mind are an important goal in themselves, but as we shall see in the next chapter, there is a wide gap between that objective and the claim that serious diseases can be defeated. Belief in the power of holism alone will not bridge that gap—what is needed is proof.

Nonetheless, the idea of the holistic approach to the patient is an immensely attractive and valuable one, and it justifiably draws towards it many patients who are fed up with being ignored by their conventional doctors, who, they feel, regard them merely as bearers of interesting diseases or "cases." In itself, holism may be one of the most important concepts in bringing conventional medicine back towards a more humane approach to patients. The idea is far too useful to be devalued by being exploited in the defence of unsupportable claims.

Unifying Hypothesis of Disease

Much of conventional medicine, unfortunately, is extremely difficult to understand. Some of it is merely complex, some of it totally obscure, some is simply *terra incognita*, some runs contrary to our intuition and common sense and some of it is just plain wrong. The welcoming committee of almost every medical school in the world tells new students that up to 50 per cent of all the medical facts taught will be shown to be wrong within ten years. Unfortunately, no one can tell the medical students in advance which 50 per cent it will be, so they have to learn it all.

Despite the efforts of doctors and scientists in the media, the practice and science of medicine still appear to the public as disturbingly heterogeneous and intellectually indigestible. Even worse, doctors sometimes seem to pride themselves on the esoteric aspects of their subject. Sometimes physicians in the media present medical information in a condescending manner. The message is almost "You're not *supposed* to understand this and you probably couldn't if you tried, but I'll give you the schoolkid's guide just to keep you quiet and show you how clever I am."

With most schools of complementary medicine, the situation is the exact opposite. Each type of alternative medicine usually has an easy-to-understand central concept of the cause of all disease and bases the therapy on remedying that fault or deficiency.

There are dozens (if not hundreds) of different concepts in alternative medicine that explain most or all of human disease. Here is one example that attributes disease to unhealthy changes in magnetic fields:

> There is now increasing evidence to support the fact that geomagnetic stress and extra low frequencies—both natural and artificial—are major causative factors in acute and chronic illnesses. Essentially there are two types of geopathic stress—the discharging field and the charging field. The discharging field can lead to energy deficiency orders [sic], such as cancer; MS; arthritis; and degenerative diseases in general, as well as fatigue. It is now thought that this type of geopathic stress is due to the presence of underground water. The charging field in some cases leads to energy excess and heart attacks, migraine headaches, etc. may result and this can be attributed to underground deposits such as coal or oil for example.[1]

Naturally, the antidote to these emanations from underground water and coal is commercially available. It is called the Reharmoniser and it "cancels out detrimental vibrations and at the same time enhances the body's ability to reharmonise itself on the mental, physical and etheric planes." The Reharmoniser consists of a small bottle of clear liquid; the owner is encouraged to keep one in each corner of every room, near any electrical devices and in the car.

> Our highly processed foods are poisoned with coal tar dyes and preservatives. The lovely green vegetables that look so inviting on the stands carry poisonous substances used as sprays intended for the extermination of bugs and pests but that find their way into the human body. ...Viewing our foods from this standpoint, it is not difficult to trace the cause of so much illness and so many degenerative diseases. The breaking down of the soil and the same deterioration found in the health of the human race have a close correlation with one another. Surely the increase of polio, heart disease, cancer—and on down the list of disease names—demonstrates the possibility of a similar origin. These are truths that are well known to our research scientists.[2]

The author of that particular pamphlet had some biological fortune on her side; at the time of writing, she was alive and well at 103 years of age. Her suggestions include washing all food in a mixture of domestic bleach and soda—but not all domestic bleaches work; in fact, only the brand Clorox is effective at a concentration of half a teaspoon per gallon water.

Another pamphlet attributes the cause of cancer to a change in the cellular electrical forces.

> Cancer is one disease with one cause. The cause is a chronic abnormal chemical work demand which affects the steady state of a differentiated cell by a definable shift in energy supply from a cross-over point (cyt,b–cyt,c) where ATP energy is being increased at the expense of a decreasing energy in (ee-H+)-1 units moving through the respiratory voltage gradient.[3]

The remedy

> lowers the voltage of the cell structure of the body by about 20%...which

is significant…because cancer cells are weak cells and lyse or convert directly to waste material when voltage is lowered…The waste material from this digestion has the appearance of raw egg whites…and the body eliminates this in any way it can…in the urine, stool, as vaginal discharge, or it may be thrown up or coughed up or eliminated in perspiration. Any all or none of these may happen.

Another author[4] has a different but equally intelligible explanation:

Cancer cells build protective jelly-like substances around themselves preventing our natural immunity system from killing them.

Again, the remedy is a plausible one:

The serum tricks the cancer cells into thinking it will help them. So cancer cells invite the serum in. The serum then dissolves the jelly-like substance and white blood cells kill the cancer. The serum then works for six months dissolving dead cancer cells.

The same serum also cures 19 other diseases, including arthritis, rheumatism, high blood pressure, diabetes, allergies, lupus, leukaemia and emphysema.

Another author, Gaston Naessens, claims to have detected a new form of universal sub-cellular particles (somatides) which he has been able to detect using his own invention, a microscope capable of achieving 30,000x magnification (compared to approximately 1800x for the conventional light microscope). Using this instrument, which he calls the Somatoscope, Naessens drew the following conclusions:[5]

1. Cellular division requires the presence of the SOMATIDE (which is either in the animal or plant domain).

2. Trephones are elaborated by the SOMATIDE.

3. The SOMATIDE is capable of polymorphism. This polymorphism is controlled by inhibitors found in the blood.

4. A deficiency of sanguine inhibitors permits the elaboration of a large quantity of trephones, which in turn lead to disorders of cellular metabolism.

5. All degenerative disorders are a consequence of these disorders.

Again, the universal nature of the root cause of human disease is immensely attractive and made even more so by Naessens's explanation that the somatide hypothesis of disease is very similar to the hukoral theories of Hippocrates and the ancients and that he has therefore proven the existence of something that has been postulated for millenia.

Many other branches of complementary medicine have similar unifying hypotheses, whether it is a macrobiotic diet, a theory of vitamin or mineral deficiency (or excess), the presence of the yeast candida or misalignment of the spine. All these hypotheses have two features in common: a single explanation of most (or all) human diseases, and a proposed form of treatment that addresses the problem at its source. Compared to the difficulties of grasping the complexities of conventional biology and medicine, these hypotheses are immensely attractive and satisfy our fundamental urge to have the complete answer presented to us in an accessible and intelligible form.

NATURAL

Many alternative therapies offer as one of their advantages the fact that they are based on some "natural" concept, technique or substance. The word "natural" has an attraction and appeal that is almost as powerful as motherhood and apple pie. The problem with "naturalness" is not that there is anything intrinsically wrong with it, but that, once again, the interpretation of the word is now so wide that it encompasses a large spectrum of concepts, many of which are fundamentally contradictory.

The central pillar of the natural schools of philosophy is that what is natural is inherently good. Conversely, what is not natural is damaging. Applied to the causation of disease, this idea implies that if humans as a species persist in behaviour that is not natural, it will produce certain problems and diseases that would not have occurred if only we had adhered to natural patterns. In this sense of the word natural—that is, those forms of behaviour for which our species has adapted structurally by means of evolution—this is often an important and sensible view. For example, if (and it is not certain but likely) we evolved from migratory anthropoids that were omnivorous and wandered about the flatlands eating a mixed diet several times a day, we might imagine that our physiology would be ill-adapted to eating large-volume high-fat meals twice a day. It might be that many years of the latter will exceed the adaptability of our biochemical homeostasis and produce certain problems. Now this does not mean that a Western diet is bound to produce problems simply *because* it is unnatural. If one wants to prove this hypothesis, one has to verify the harmful effects of Western diet and then show that the parts of the world in which the diet more closely resembles the diet of our earliest ancestors are free of these problems.

So far so good: if you know what problems our species has solved during its evolution, this may give you insight into understanding diseases caused by our contemporary life styles. This is clearly a useful and attractive way of looking at things. However, the central concept of "what is natural is inherently good" is often extended much further to support every variety of remedy—and this creates the problems. The mere fact of being natural or derived from natural materials does not mean that a medicine or remedy is essentially better than its counterpart. It is true that aspirin was derived from natural sources (willow bark) as was digitalis (foxglove), quinine, some anti-cancer drugs (vincristine from the periwinkle, etoposide from the mandrake root and taxol from the Pacific yew) and that these have been shown to be active drugs. On the other hand, laetrile, a frequently used "anti-cancer" alternative remedy, is equally natural (it is derived from apricot pits) but is inactive, as are Essiac and many others. What makes a drug useful is its effectiveness, not its naturalness. The same is true of side effects; if two drugs are equally effective but one of them will produce fewer side effects, then it would be advisable to use that one—whether or not it is derived from natural products. Once again, the origin of the substance tells you nothing about its actions—therapeutic or inadvertent.

Furthermore, within complementary medicine—and even more within the commercial companies that follow and benefit from its popularity and accessibility—the concept of naturalness has been greatly over-used and frequently exploited. For example, wheat is natural (though only partly, because it has been genetically modulated in cultivation). Grinding wheat, on the other hand, is totally unnatural and baking it is even more so. Hence all bread is unnatural, and there is no difference in the naturalness of brown and white bread. There is, on the other hand, a great difference between them in fibre content. Our acceptance of the health-giving virtue of fibre depends on the evidence from studies that correlate high-fibre diets with low incidence of diseases (gallstones, diverticulitis, some cancers and so on). It does not depend simply on philosophical thoughts about natural brown bread.

This same analysis of the method of processing should also be applied to drugs. Many herbs—despite their naturalness of origin—go through processes that are far from natural before they reach the patient in the form of medicines. There is nothing natural, for example, in doing what homeopaths do and diluting a herb extract 2000 million million times while systematically shaking the tube in a special vibrating device.

We are not attacking (or defending) the concept of naturalness in itself. It's just that whether a remedy is natural or not may have no relevance to its usefulness—it may be natural and useless or natural and useful (or synthetic and useful or synthetic and useless). The same is true of anything one cares to think of—including diseases; for instance, as someone once pointed out, the smallpox virus and the tapeworm are both natural—and so is cancer. In fact, cancer cells are not only natural to the species, they are natural to the host—they are the patient's own cells that have simply lost their ability to respond to control signals. They are so natural that the patient's immune system does not even recognize them as foreign, which is how cancers manage to grow.

The situation was different in the past, when combatting the forces of nature seemed to be a major achievement. Nature, complete with its plagues and predators, was seen then as "red in tooth and claw" and it is only recently that we have come to think of it as a healing force, inherently nurturing and kind. Neither of these simplistic generalizations is accurate, of course, but it is worth remembering that any talk of the kindness of nature rather depends on your viewpoint; for instance, many people are alive today—one of the authors of this book (R.B.) included—whom nature would clearly prefer to be dead. Inherited diseases (autoimmune conditions, in this example) can kill, and if the patient dies before having children, the genetic pool of the species will be steadily strengthened by that culling. If the patient survives and reproduces, the faulty genes— admittedly diluted by his or her partner—will pollute the gene pool. Thus nature (if it can be personified as a force), in being kind to the species as a whole, has to be very cruel to the individual and usually favours the death of the weak specimen for the good of the herd. One's interpretation of the kindness of nature thus depends very materially on whether one is a member of the healthy herd or the sick subgroup.

TRADITIONAL

Alternative medicine often attracts people because it professes to be "traditional." It seems to be part of the contradictory nature of our species that we admire both the most modern trends in any area and also the most traditional, rather like the extremely expensive Japanese electronic piano that has been programmed to feel and sound exactly like a concert Steinway.

Perhaps the major primary attraction of a traditional remedy is that "it has been around for years, hundreds of thousands of people have used it and they cannot be totally mistaken so it must be worth a try." There is merit in this line of reasoning—for instance, it is probably a relatively safe assumption that the remedy is free from major toxic effects. Traditional remedies are, on the whole, non-toxic for the simple reason that particularly nasty remedies do not get passed on down the generations—a form of almost-natural selection.

However, there seems to be an even deeper and more significant reason for liking tradition. When we are threatened by illness, one of the most prominent feelings is that of isolation; patients feel isolated from everyone else by their illness; they feel alone and vulnerable. Taking a remedy that has been used for generations gives a small but perceptible sense of community with other patients and of belonging, even though the association is with nameless and faceless people who have been down the same path. There is no great harm in this at all, but it needs to be stressed once more that the mere traditional origin of a remedy does not tell you anything about its effectiveness. Like naturalness, the tradition of a remedy tells you only about its provenance—that in itself may be of comfort but may bear no relationship to its effectiveness.

In addition to creating an approving attitude to the treatment, the label "traditional" lends an aura to the healer that conventional doctors may not have.

There are many examples of this aura, but one that illustrates most of the relevant features is the story of René Caisse, a Canadian proponent of the herbal remedy Essiac. Caisse's story had a large number of charismatic elements to it.[6] She came from the Bracebridge area of Ontario and was trained as a nurse. When she was 33 years old, she met an 80-year-old woman who had previously had advanced cancer of the breast. Rather than face conventional surgery, this woman had taken a herbal tea from an old Indian man in the local mining camp. Her tumours shrank, leaving scars only. Twenty years later she told her story to René Caisse and gave her the old Indian's recipe for the tea. Caisse first used the tea to treat her aunt (who was said to have stomach cancer and to have less than six months to live), and then started treating other cancer patients. Caisse's aunt went on to survive a further 21 years, and Caisse became a national and international wonder, treating thousands of cancer patients with her herbal tea, now called Essiac (Caisse spelled backwards). She never revealed the secret recipe to the government of Canada, nor to the largest and most illustrious cancer centres in the United States. She was revered by her patients and co-workers alike and died at the age of 90.

It is not difficult to see the intuitive attraction of that story and how comforting the various elements are to patients who are bewildered and confused by modern conventional medicine and its high-tech soullessness. Essiac is redolent of our human origins and the traditional roots that we all fear we've lost. It not only promises cures based on decades of experience, but it also offers a fundamental sense of connectedness and continuity. Even for patients who have absolutely nothing in common with the Indians of Ontario, the story of Essiac induces a profound sense of nostalgia and of belonging.

By contrast, conventional doctors seem to lack all these reassuring elements and are seen as proponents of a style of medicine that is continually changing, innovating and using new technology. There is a popular perception that alternative practitioners are in some way guardians of a kind of casket of traditional medical practices, to whom the keys have been passed by previous generations of healers. But such an image is a mirage. There is a stronger argument for continuity of practice among successive generations of conventional medical practitioners than there is for the disparate and sometimes contradictory disciplines that make up alternative medicine. Far from being guardians of anything at all, many alternative healers have no formal training and no contact with earlier generations of healers.

EXOTIC

Another example of the paradoxical reactions that we humans exhibit when threatened by illness is the attraction of the traditional and the simultaneous appeal of the exotic. We are using the word "exotic" in the narrow sense of "originating from another culture." Clearly while most Westerners regard Ayurvedic medicine as exotic, in Bangladesh it is the most accessible and cheapest medical care, whereas an intravenous infusion of saline (mundane treatment in Western hospitals) is regarded with a respect verging on awe.

So why are we attracted to exotic and trans-cultural remedies? The answer seems to lie in the hope that other peoples—and particularly their ancestors—stumbled upon the answers to mysteries that we have not solved. We hope that early in the civilization of China (or India or Peru) the ancients discovered a remedy or perfected a body of knowledge that they passed on exclusively to their own descendants and that was never discovered in our own culture. Sometimes this turns out to be correct. Perhaps the most famous example is curare. Curare is derived from plants of the genus *Strychnos* and is used as an arrow-tip poison by natives of South America to paralyze their animal prey. It achieved wide usage in the West only in the 1930s, when the analysis of its chemical structure not only provided the basis for synthetic muscle relaxants in anaesthetics, but also facilitated major discoveries in the physiology of nerve conduction.

But curare is the exception. There are many other folk remedies with no demonstrable effect that have been taken up on a massive scale predominantly on account of the exoticism of their origins. Perhaps the current use of ginseng is the most recent example, but there are many others, including tiger balm and royal jelly, both of which have long traditions in Chinese medicine.

The appeal of the exotic may well derive from the more general appeal of the unfamiliar. As we explore the power of belief in affecting how the ill body responds to different remedies, we'll see how in conventional medicine as well as in alternative therapies, the strange, unusual, abnormal or attention-getting aspects of therapies contribute perhaps 30 per cent of their overall effectiveness. A flower scent extracted from a plant picked on one specific day of the year in a particular location is more exotic than a bubble-packed pill manufactured by a major American conglomerate and may therefore have a different effect.

There is another aspect of illness in which exoticism may play an important part. Illness can be a mysterious and exotic invasion of one's inner space, like a dragon. Perhaps it is true to say that when humans are confronted by the dragons of illness, they look for a St. George to defend them—and the exotically mysterious stranger from another culture just might turn out to be the St. George that they are hoping for. This is even more likely to be true when the local knight is not St. George but simple Dr. George and is not encountered astride a white charger but, at best, is seated behind a big shiny desk with a fat prescription pad.

Significance

Many, perhaps most, alternative therapists give to their patients a greater sense of personal significance than they get from doctors.

The inevitable "mass production" aspect of a modern medical care system leads to a need to categorize people in terms very different from the way they normally see themselves. This is particularly worrying for patients—sick people or those who believe themselves to be sick—because losing the sense of oneself as a significant being is one of the most frightening aspects of falling unwilling victim to a failure of the body and becoming ill. Not only is identity lost, but with it the significance of being this particular person. An ill person becomes a "victim of colitis" or "a cancer sufferer" or an "AIDS patient" or "a case of malaria" or "an abdominal emergency" or "the cardiac arrest on Ward 4."

In terms of medical care, all these labels are to some extent justified and are certainly not intended primarily to strip the person of identity and significance. It is important to have some form of instantly recognizable label so that health care professionals know what is expected of them in providing the appropriate services. The medical needs of a person with a fractured femur are obviously quite different from those of a person with renal failure, and the professionals require labels in order to transmit large amounts of information to each other quickly and efficiently. If an ambulance attendant radios ahead to an emergency department with the words "diabetic coma," the staff of the department will be ready to use intravenous infusions, insulin, central venous pressure monitoring, potassium supplements, hourly glucose and electrolyte measurements and so on. If the ambulance attendant only said, "We're bringing in Mr. Jones, a gentle animal-loving Capricorn whose life up to now has been blessed with good karma," nobody would know how urgent the situation was or what to prepare. Obviously, then, diagnostic labelling works well in crises. However, the disadvantage of diagnostic labels is that when there is no crisis, too often (in conventional medicine) the label is all that is used and the "Mr. Jones" part is forgotten.

But in highlighting the loss of significance we are not talking merely of depersonalization. The anonymity and the "faceless number" syndrome of hospital patients is certainly important (as we have mentioned above), but we are dealing here with the threat of the loss of personhood in the illness and that is more than the loss of identity. If a person is found to have a disease, that disease will broadly be the same for each person, in the sense that blood samples, urine samples, pancreatic biopsy and so on would be indistinguishable in the type of pathology they showed. But the *meaning* of the illness for that person will be very different—Mr. Jones's diabetes is not the same as Mrs. Wilson's diabetes in the way that it affects them individually. Both of them may require the same daily dose of insulin and both of them may require monthly follow-up visits, regular blood tests or urine testing, but, in addition to that, each patient is a person to whom the illness means something. The meaning of an illness to the individual who has it is an important concept.

We must be clear about our use of the word "meaning" here. In this context, we use the word to indicate what the illness itself means to the patient (the *extrinsic* meaning of the illness) as opposed to the meaning of that illness in general (that is, the meaning that the illness always brings to every patient—the *intrinsic* meaning). In fact, the idea that diseases have any intrinsic and predetermined meanings at all is a dubious one. Thus we do *not* subscribe to the view that many illnesses are caused by the individual's personal characteristics (aside from behavioural factors such as smoking causing lung cancer, drinking causing liver damage and so on), and we do not accept the view that, for example, breast cancer afflicts only those women for whom it is a fitting and appropriate solution to some personal problem or an escape for unresolved anger and so on. Currently many people—including many complementary practitioners—do believe that most diseases are largely predetermined by personality and attitude and thus do have an intrinsic meaning ("You got this disease because you were never angry enough"), particularly when the diagnosis is cancer.

One of the questions patients most often ask the doctor or healer when they fall ill is "Why me?" or "Why did this happen?" Alternative healers, unlike conventional doctors, are rarely lost for an answer. Contrast the bleakness of "I'm afraid we just don't know" or "These things are really just random" with "Your chakras are unbalanced because of a recent spiritual upset," "You've been eating too many yin foods and not enough yang" or "You've been bottling up your feelings and we're going to have to find ways of letting them out." Apart from anything else, a persuasive explanation offers hope of some kind of cure, whereas if the doctor doesn't know why something struck you and not your next-door neighbour, how can you believe in his ability to treat? Once again, as with "tradition," "naturalness" and "exoticism," patients can sometimes infer a message about the *effectiveness* of a treatment from a characteristic that has nothing to do with effectiveness. In fact, there are many examples of diseases whose origins or causes are unknown but which can be successfully treated by doctors, just as there are plenty of diseases about which a lot is known but which still cannot be successfully treated.

Whatever the cause of the disease, the person who suffers from it is threatened with the loss of personal significance unless someone helps him or her rediscover it. Conventional doctors are rarely good at helping the patient with that process; complementary practitioners usually are.

David and Goliath

Another factor that makes complementary medicine attractive is the fact that most forms of it are simple and low-tech compared with the large expensive apparatus and paraphernalia of conventional medicine. In some respects, patients identify the complementary practitioners as plucky little Davids facing the Goliaths of establishment medicine. This is particularly obvious when conventional medical establishments (colleges or medical associations) try to condemn or ban some branch of complementary medicine. Those complementary practitioners may not have been perceived as Davids until they face the might of Goliath-style behaviour.

There are many reasons for this widespread sympathy with complementary medicine and the desire to see conventional medicine rebuffed. Conventional doctors spend five to seven years in their undergraduate training, perhaps another two in general training and then (depending on their career choice) up to six or seven more years in specialty training and (often) research. During this process they may acquire several higher degrees that entitle them to trail half the alphabet after their names. They are also likely to acquire high social status and high salaries (depending on their country of practice). Quite often they are proud of their achievements (sometimes justifiably) and of the knowledge that they have worked so hard to acquire. It is that pride that irks both patients and public if it becomes too visible. For instance, in the United States, the National Cancer Institute has an annual budget (currently) of about $2 billion. It would appeal to the human sympathies of most of us if the cure for cancer were discovered not within those tall and expensive walls, but in the front room of a little guy down the road who boiled up some herbs according to an ancient recipe.

An example of this process occurred in the 1960s when in many countries it was believed that Dr. Josef Issels of Switzerland had discovered the cure for leukaemia (and perhaps other cancers) by removing the tonsils, bad teeth and any other foci of infection, and then administering a variety of treatments, including fever-producing materials and (apparently) ozone. This approach became extremely popular. Many of Issels's patients felt that the central philosophy was so obvious that the conventional cancer physicians had simply overlooked it. Dr. Issels's clinic in Bavaria was later shut down after investigations by the medical authorities, but in many respects that closure was regarded as the medical equivalent of martyrdom and, if anything, enhanced his reputation and the faith that patients had in his methods.

The same thing happened more recently in Athens where Dr. Hariton Alivizatos has been treating 3000 cancer patients a year, with apparently high success rates and no adverse effects.[7] His career has also been dogged by persecution from conventional authorities. By his own account, even his medical graduation was withheld because the authorities wanted him to reveal the formula of his secret serum and was awarded only after a court battle. The Greek Medical Association later accused him of advertising and withdrew his license—a decision that was subsequently reversed after a further lengthy court battle.

Another famous example is the work of Dr. Royal Rife (1888-1971). His life's work is detailed in *The Cancer Cure That Worked—Fifty Years of Suppression*.[8] Rife reportedly discovered that all cancers are caused by a virus (detected only by his own special microscope, which was the most powerful in the world and magnified 17,000 diameters). Rife and colleagues established the world's first successful cancer clinic in 1934 and reportedly reversed cancers in human patients by killing the viruses. However, the methodology was so unconventional and so challenging to the authorities that, it is said, his work was suppressed and covered up.

But perhaps one of the best recent examples of how persecution can be seen as evidence of the rectitude and far-sightedness of the victim is the story of the trial of Gaston Naessens.

Gaston Naessens is the French biologist we mentioned above who is now established in Quebec, Canada. He claims to have invented the Somatoscope, an extraordinary microscope with which he has identified sub-cellular particles that are the cause of most human diseases and are virtually indestructible, being resistant to temperatures of 200°C and massive doses of radiation.

Over the years, Naessens produced several different remedies, his most recent being 714-X (named for the seventh and fourteenth letters of the alphabet, which are his initials, the X representing the twenty-fourth letter—he was born in 1924). When 714-X was subjected to analysis by the Health Protection Branch of the Health and Welfare Department of the government of Canada, it was found to consist of camphor, ammonium chloride and nitrate, sodium chloride, ethanol and water.[9]

Naessens, although not a physician, treated many patients, including over a thousand cases of cancer and over a dozen patients with AIDS.

Naessens was arrested and tried in 1989 over the death of a patient with breast cancer who, it was alleged, might have been effectively treated by conventional therapy had she not taken Naessens's therapy. The trial created widespread public interest and debate and provided a major focus for the supporters and followers of Naessens. For them the entire trial was akin to a form of martyrdom that in itself proved the veracity of Naessen's claims ("If there wasn't something in it, why are the authorities making all this fuss?"). Naessens was acquitted.

The trial consolidated and focused support for Naessens and is analyzed in triumphant detail in a book *The Galileo of the Microscope*.[10] The trial itself fills more than two-thirds of the book, reducing biology and biography almost to incidental notes. There is no doubt that persecution by the authorities is perceived by believers as a badge of credibility ("He must be a true David if he induces this response from the Goliaths"), and the attempt to suppress or stop the complementary practitioner from continuing the treatment moves the debate away from a discussion of any truth or validity of the work itself into a web of legalese and litigation procedure.

JUSTICE

There is another deep-seated sense that is stimulated by complementary medicine, and that is a sense of justice or equity. This is particularly true of those branches of complementary medicine in which the patient's personality or mind-set is thought to play an important part in the causation of the disease and in its progress. Perhaps the best example in recent times is that of the philosophy of Dr. Bernie Siegel. Dr. Siegel is an oncological (cancer) surgeon at Yale who noted certain personality characteristics of patients who did better than he expected. He termed these patients "exceptional cancer patients" or *E-CaPs* and identified the personality traits that improved their prognosis as a will to survive and an ability to achieve inner peace and to be kind and forgiving to themselves. Although adopting these personal attitudes is not guaranteed to improve the prognosis, Dr. Siegel's books are filled with advice on how to achieve these states and thus improve the chances of survival.

This philosophy has a tremendously powerful appeal, and a major constituent of that appeal is justice and fairness. If the Siegel characteristics do determine survival, then only the people who *really* want to survive will do so. The people who fall by the wayside will fall because they did not want to survive enough. It does not matter if you are the richest woman or man in the world, and whether you have access to the most expensive and best treatment, if in your heart you do not have the survivor instinct, then your chances will not be so good. On the other hand, whatever your station in the material world—however little a guy (or presumably doll) you are, if you really want to make it through, you will. There are other reasons that this view of disease is so attractive, and we shall deal with those in a later chapter.

However, at present there is no evidence that survivor characteristics affect the survival of cancer patients at all (though interestingly enough there is some evidence that good social bonding and support from friends and group therapy might[11]). Nevertheless, Dr. Siegel's ideas have stimulated tremendous enthusiasm in the United States, perhaps in part because Dr Siegel's world would be a much fairer one if it were true.

The list of factors above—from energy fields to exoticism—highlights, we believe, some of the things that have contributed to the popularity of alternative medicine in recent years. They centre on a set of beliefs about these therapies, beliefs that are not necessarily correct but that get the patient through the door to the healer. But these therapies have other characteristics that actually supply something special to the patient, regardless of whether the therapy is truly exotic, natural, traditional or holistic.

6. Practical Plusses and Minuses

---

*Nobody in his or her right mind ever wants
to hear a doctor say, "Nothing can be done."*

Plusses of Complementary Medicine

When it comes to the practice of the healer-patient interaction, the physical and psychological details of the patient's visit to the doctor or healer, there are many attractive features of the complementary practitioner's *modus operandi*, and a few somewhat unattractive or even distasteful aspects of the conventional doctor's usual methods.

Hope

David Prescott, a 48-year-old Englishman, flew to a laetrile clinic in Tijuana, Mexico, in order to try complementary medicine. His cancer of the bowel had been diagnosed two years previously. In the last month or so, he had begun to lose weight and to feel uncomfortable in the upper right side of his abdomen. A recent scan had shown that there were secondaries from the bowel cancer in his liver. When asked what had prompted him to come to Mexico, he replied, "The doctors in England said there was nothing they could do for me, and at least these people here are willing to have a go." He underwent a two-week course of therapy, which included visualization sessions, treatment with laetrile and coffee enemas.

With potentially fatal diseases, the attraction of complementary medicine is easy to see. No normal person wants to die alone. Sadly, it is one of the failings of conventional medicine that, by and large, conventional doctors are not as good at looking after the dying as they

100

could be, and some patients in the conventional medical system feel that, as they face death, they are on their own. Of course, matters have changed considerably in the last three decades, and there are now many doctors, special units and hospices where high-quality care of the dying is practised. Despite these encouraging and important developments, however, many doctors still are better at looking after the potentially curable than the incurable; they feel ill-equipped to deal with and support patients whom they cannot cure and whose death is expected. This was the case with the doctor looking after David Prescott. As a surgeon, the doctor was a superb—perhaps brilliant—technician whose skill and dexterity had made him famous. However, he was not so accomplished when the disease proved more powerful than his therapeutic skills, and he had told David that there was "nothing more that could be done" (or David recalled it that way).

Almost certainly, David's surgeon meant something slightly different. He probably meant that further surgery was futile and that nothing more could be done *to cure the disease*. Doctors frequently say "Nothing can be done" without, unfortunately, making it clear that they are talking about the disease, not the patient in person. Frequently, that statement is really a disclaimer, almost an apology. Doctors in this situation often would like to say something like "This disease is unstoppable. I have done as much as I can; please don't blame me as things get worse." However, a statement like that sounds personal and indicates the doctor's own human emotions, which, in general, conventional doctors are discouraged in their training from revealing.

David Prescott felt that he had been abandoned, and abandonment at that particular time of crisis—when secondaries had just been detected—was the most crushing blow he had ever experienced. He perceived it as a brush-off and, not unnaturally, cast about looking for someone who would offer something, anything.

Of course, not all patients who go to complementary practitioners have a life-threatening or terminal illness. But their situation exemplifies—albeit in an extreme form—two of the main reasons for which patients go to complementary practitioners: for hope and for support.

It was always one of the basic tenets of medical school education that a good doctor "never takes away all hope from the patient." Unfortunately, very few senior physicians ever taught their juniors how to talk to patients truthfully without apparently removing hope. As a result, many doctors grew up thinking that the only way they could avoid taking away hope was by avoiding all conversations about the future so simply refuse to be drawn into difficult dialogue with the patient. Complementary practitioners, on the other hand, operate without those constraints. Generally, complementary practitioners are not expected (by their patients) to have such a detailed knowledge of the progress and prognosis of the diseases or conditions they may treat. Their patients often do not therefore expect a detailed forecast from them and indeed may well have already received that from their conventional doctors. Unconfined by the need to gaze into what might be a grim crystal ball, the complementary practitioners usually find it relatively easy to offer hope. Furthermore, they are usually not as conscious of statistics as conventional doctors are (and are obliged to be).

When a cancer specialist sees a patient with, let us say, a type of lung cancer called small-cell carcinoma, the doctor knows that five years after diagnosis, 19 out of every 20 patients will have died—5 per cent will survive. If a patient asks, "Will I make it to five years?" a good (and honest) doctor will feel an obligation to be truthful and is likely to say that there is a chance of that happening but it is a relatively slim one. Obviously, the answer will be (or should be) delivered as gently as possible, continuing the dialogue with the patient, responding to his or her reactions and offering continued support. However, it would be unfair, possibly unethical—and would not provide the patient with the information for which he or she is asking—if the doctor answered, "I don't see why you shouldn't."

Usually, complementary practitioners are not bound by those particular kind of ethical guidelines. A complementary practitioner when asked "Will I make it to five years?" might easily answer, "I know many in your situation who did" or "If you want to enough, perhaps you will." Both those answers are literally correct—particularly in the first case, if the doctor had seen such a large number of patients that 5 per cent of them was "many," and in the second case provided that the word "perhaps" is carefully included.

Although patients are likely to hear more hopeful responses from complementary practitioners, they are also less likely to hear what David Prescott heard: "Nothing can be done." When conventional doctors say that, there is an implication of "I'm afraid you will just have to accept this and live with it the way it is." In other words, some conventional doctors regard the end of therapeutic endeavour as the end of what they can do for the patient. By contrast, the absence of an effective therapy does not necessarily worry many complementary practitioners. Although many of them will administer therapy of one type or another in the hope that it may cause improvement, few of them become upset if it does not work. For many such practitioners, patients with chronic, unchanging or progressive diseases make up a high proportion of their practice, and continuing to look after them even with diminishing hope of effective therapy is a major part of their attractiveness.

Finally, it is worth recalling that the words "despair" and "desperation" are both derived from the same ancient root and mean "loss of hope." The absence of all hope is a dreadful state and the urge to go anywhere that offers some hope is, literally, the urge of desperation. It remains a criticism of conventional doctors that, by and large, the profession is not good at offering hope of good symptom control, of support, of understanding and of continuity when the hope of cure has gone. It is for that reason that many patients equate a doctor's "no hope of cure" with a final and dismissive "no hope of care" which is tantamount to no hope at all.

Support

Both healers and patients use the word "support" freely and frequently but it seems difficult to get a precise definition of what constitutes support in the context of personal health. Although we all may be talking about something slightly different, there is a general central core upon which everyone can agree. Certainly, when people feel ill, support is something that they want and need, and when support is lacking, patients are almost always dissatisfied.

As a rough approximation, the following are probably the most important components of support.

Time: One of the points most commonly noted by patients of conventional doctors (usually as a criticism, but occasionally as a mark of admiration) is how busy the doctor seems to be. In family practice, the visits are often six minutes or less; in hospital practice, the doctor may be paged several times during a conversation or may have to rush away to a meeting or conference. One of the side effects of this "busy-ness" is that the patient is constantly being reminded that she or he is less important than the incoming phone call or the meeting. Strangely enough, conventional doctors are taught very little about time management (or people management) at medical school. Dealing with priority calls and making the patient they are with feel significant is something few medical students understand; their counterparts in the world of commerce have a far more thorough training in how to make the customer feel significant.

By contrast, most complementary practitioners are experts at the mechanics of time management and giving patients the sensation that the healer's time belongs to the patient. An air of being unhurried and unflustered is common in most complementary settings and is much prized.

Personal involvement: Support for the patient also has to be personal—it has to be tailored to fit the needs and idiosyncrasies of the individual patient. Support does not seem to be transmissible in a pre-packaged form (the psychotherapeutic equivalent of "have a nice day"). For a patient to feel supported, it is important that the healer indicate that she or he is treating this person as an individual and is aware of the particular features and agenda that this individual brings to the relationship. Again, conventional doctors do not learn how to do this, whereas most complementary practitioners are either intuitively skilled at this, or learn it rapidly in their apprenticeship.

Another component of the personal involvement is dependent on continuity of care. A patient who sees a different (perhaps a junior) doctor at each visit (more usual in hospitals than in family practice) soon feels depersonalized. On the other hand, a patient who is greeted by name by a healer who remembers his or her story without needing to flip through the case file will feel more personally integrated into that medical service. An interesting point is that as the field of complementary medicine expands and takes in more trainees, patients are more likely to be seen by new and junior personnel, and similar complaints of discontinuity and anonymity are beginning to be heard in the larger complementary medicine centres.

Other interpersonal skills: Another area in which, until recently, conventional doctors have been weak is that of interpersonal skills, particularly interview skills. These include how to (and when to) touch patients, how to deal with a patient who cries or is angry and so on. Nowadays skills such as these are being incorporated into medical school curricula, but until a few years ago this area was one in which most complementary practitioners had a considerable lead over conventional doctors. It might be too extreme to suggest that alternative healers take up their calling to cure *patients* while doctors become doctors to cure *diseases*. But working as a member of the medical profession embodies a mixture of pure science, detective work, discovery and fame, as well as the opportunity to help ordinary people with their ordinary complaints, and so it would not be surprising if some people who became doctors were ill-equipped to care, nurture and explain but made exceptional pathologists, heads of research units or epidemiologists.

Empathy: Empathy is, in essence, the quality of personal caring extended into the realm of emotions. In medical (and psychiatric) language, the word "empathy" means identifying and acknowledging the emotions that the patient is experiencing. It does not mean that the healer has to feel the same emotion himself or herself ("You do not have to cry or bleed with every patient"). Empathy—in the form of empathic response—is a technique that can be easily learned and taught. However, unless empathy is taught as a specific technique, many conventional doctors are uncomfortable in dealing with a patient's emotions. Some see nothing strange about the fact that, in spite of a dislike of sick people, they have chosen a profession where they are likely to come into daily contact with them.

Most complementary practitioners are intuitively empathic—and perhaps self-selected on that basis, whereas it is a quality unlooked for in candidates applying to conventional medical schools.

Acceptance: The empathic response is the means by which a healer may indicate that she or he *acknowledges* the patient's emotions. However, there is another element that adds even more support to the interaction: that is the healer's *acceptance* of the patient's problems. Conventional doctors are taught to interpret the patient's symptoms; for example, a pain in the heart region brought on by spicy foods may not be a heart attack but oesophagitis. In fact, clinical medicine requires a high degree of sophisticated interpretation in order to organize the appropriate tests and treatment. Interpretation by its very nature implies translation—in this case from the patient's perception of the problem, to the doctor's knowledge of the medical condition ("You say it's your heart, but I know it's your oesophagus"). There is nothing intrinsically wrong with this process; in fact, it is essential for the process of diagnosis. The problem is that patients require something else as well. They require the healer's acceptance of their symptoms, and, more importantly, acceptance of their own reactions (fears, anxieties and so on) to those symptoms. In other words, they require the healer to acknowledge the existence of what they are experiencing (even if it signifies something else in terms of disease) and of their feelings. This can be achieved relatively easily, but unfortunately most doctors have not been shown how to do it. Hence they appear to be satisfied at having made the correct diagnosis and are apparently uninterested in what concerns the patient most—the symptoms themselves and what they mean to him or her. Complementary practitioners generally have a personal style diametrically opposed to that of conventional doctors. Usually, acceptance is the first response with which they greet the patient's problem list, and it is very much appreciated as part of the support.

These, then, seem to be the main components of that quality which most of us recognize as support and which many patients feel they are more likely to get from complementary practitioners than from some conventional doctors. It is worth stressing that whether a patient feels that she or he is getting support from a person does not necessarily depend on that person providing her or his medical care. Healers with all the above qualities may not be supervising the patient's care, and, in some respects, it is almost easier to offer support and hope to a patient if you are not the person responsible for seeing them every day or week and having to tell them bad news or hear that the treatment is not working.

Control

Loss of control, like loss of significance, is one of the most fearsome aspects of being ill. It usually begins with the disease (few of us will be able to control the onset, timing and progress of our illnesses, and usually we are surprised involuntarily by all three), and it often continues with the treatment. Unfortunately, most conventional doctors have not yet learned how to remedy that feeling by sharing control of the medical situation with the patient. Doctors usually assume complete control over all aspects of "the case"—which may be entirely appropriate in an acute emergency when there is little time for discussion, but is inappropriate in the great majority of medical consultations when there is ample time and opportunity. In fact, the need for control by the doctor in acute situations is reinforced by professional regulations and by laws that punish doctors for mismanaging an emergency or a treatable or curable condition. Unfortunately, many conventional doctors have become a little dazzled by the "acute emergency" mode of behaviour and as a profession they have not yet fully realized that many patients do not have acute emergencies but do have chronic or incurable conditions in which their participation could be encouraged and in which their opinions and references for treatment may have relevance.

Certainly things are changing steadily, but doctor control is still a common phenomenon (perhaps more so in Britain than in the United States or Canada). As a result, patients in conventional medicine systems often feel that they have no control over most aspects of their care, whereas in complementary medicine they are involved as active participants. It is as if complementary medicine offers them the choices available to consumers in a supermarket, whereas conventional medicine makes them feel as if they are the products on the shelves, labelled, packaged and handled impersonally.

Perhaps the classic example of the way in which complementary medicine appears to offer control to the patient is diet. There are a very large number of diets offered by complementary practitioners for food allergies, arthritic complaints, headaches and conditions of every degree of seriousness up to and including cancer. There is very little objective evidence that a change of diet is helpful in any condition except major food allergies, but even so such diets are adopted extremely widely. One of the main reasons for this is that the diet is one of the few things that remains permanently under the patient's control. Whether it exerts any beneficial effect by being a form of displaced occupational therapy or not, it is an example of the powerful attraction of returning control to the patient.

As we shall see later, there are techniques that any professionals can use to help the patient regain control—and that should be employed much more widely in conventional medicine. But at present there is still a widespread feeling that participation in control is something more easily available in complementary practice than in conventional medicine.

Non-toxic

A new word achieved wide currency and fame about 30 years ago. Although the phenomenon had been around for centuries, it did not have a name and it hadn't been well-known or publicly discussed. The word was "iatrogenic" and it was almost invariably used in the phrase "iatrogenic diseases" or, more politely, "iatrogenic problems." The word means "caused by a doctor" ("iatro" is the same root as in the word "psychiatrist"—mind-doctor), and it refers to the fact that doctors either by direct intervention (surgery, for example) or by the use of powerful drugs often create new problems for the patient while they solve (or try to solve) the old ones. In fact, "quite often" may be understatement—various studies have suggested that iatrogenic problems are the main or contributory cause in at least 10 per cent of hospital admissions, and in some series nearly 30 per cent. The image of "the fireman who starts the fires" has unfortunately stuck—and is firmly attached to both the medical profession and the manufacturers of the drugs and devices that the profession uses.

It really reached public consciousness with the thalidomide disaster. The ironies of modern medicine have never been displayed more acutely than when a drug that was prescribed for morning sickness in pregnancy turned out to cause major deformities in the fetuses of the pregnant women. The combination of "trivial" use with horrifying side effect seemed to exemplify the risks of modern drugs and the commercialism of the pharmaceutical industry. The many highly publicized cases that followed thalidomide have just reinforced the belief that if a drug causes a single major side effect or adverse reaction, particularly death, the manufacturers must accept that it has no use in modern medicine and take it off the market. This view is reinforced by the sight of a sick or injured person being awarded large amounts of money from a drug company, despite the company's ability to pay for the best lawyers.

Certainly in some cases, the drug companies have dragged their feet in reporting harmful effects, and in a few cases it seems likely that they suppressed important information in an attempt to consolidate their share of the market. On the other hand, there has been hype and hyper-hype on both sides. Some cases have attracted more than their fair share of publicity due to the energy and media-management abilities of the patients or support groups. Sometimes the mere threat of a several-million-dollar lawsuit has caused companies to withdraw a product and settle out of court, despite the absence of any firm evidence of harm. Yet despite any exaggeration on either side, there is no doubt that powerful drugs (or devices or operations) can cause powerful side effects. When the disease for which the intervention is prescribed is serious, the risk may be worth taking. When the original problem is less serious, the chance of major side effects may simply be too high a price to pay.

This raises an important question—one that has never been adequately discussed: Is there enough justification for the large-scale production of drugs for minor complaints? There are clearly two sides to the question. On the one hand, patients with minor troublesome symptoms might be glad of relief, and pharmaceutical companies would be glad to sell large quantities of a drug. On the other hand, if it happens that there are major side effects (no matter how rare), then the cost-benefit balance for the individual patient becomes extremely tricky. Clearly this is an unresolvable issue—particularly since the people who most want drugs for minor symptoms may not be the people who are most easily moved to sue pharmaceutical companies. However, it does seem that the large market for drugs is not entirely due to the marketing strategies of drug manufacturers. We would suggest that there has been complicity, and that the public has not always been seduced by cold-hearted greedy company men, but that there has been a relationship of mutual interest and (occasionally) fascination. The public has been attracted by the idea that every deviation from a feeling of full health could be fixed by the appropriate drug, and the manufacturers have been equally attracted by the idea of providing the chemical wherewithal. Perhaps, as is the case with so much of illness, the problem is partly that the patient has difficulty in finding somebody who will listen. As we say many times in this book, the severity of many common symptoms varies with the patient's view of their significance. Many symptoms are more bearable once they have been acknowledged and accepted by a healer, and perhaps some drug-taking (for minor degrees of worry or unhappiness, and minor problems in getting to sleep) succeeds because of something in the healer-patient interaction rather than in a tablet. It is quite possible that a person feeling unhappy or worried has no ready audience or confidante to discuss it with and goes to the doctor in lieu of anyone else. However, once the person has decided to go the doctor, he or she then has to behave like a patient—and make the central part of the transaction the symptoms instead of the cause of the unhappiness. Once someone has entered the patient role, the doctor may feel obliged to enter the doctor role—in which the prescription seems to have an important function. Hence, both the patient and the doctor may become locked into a transaction that neither of them really wants, with an outcome that suits neither of them. It is not difficult to imagine that the patient's dissatisfaction in being given a tablet instead of listening time may be reflected in the appearance of side effects. Symptoms are always harder to bear in an atmosphere of disaffection.

This is not the appropriate forum to debate the fundamental rights and the wrongs of this issue, but it is quite clear that there is, at present among large sections of the population, an atmosphere of increasing disenchantment with drugs for non-essential purposes. The lawsuits and the human-interest stories highlight the drawbacks of conventional therapy, and the absence of toxicity in most complementary medicine becomes more and more of an attraction.

The public image, then, of the sort of drugs that are handed out by conventional doctors is one that is bedevilled by issues of toxicity. Both side effects (predictable accompaniments to treatments) and adverse reactions (unpredictable responses to treatment in a few individuals) have become less tolerated by the public as the effects have increased. (Although, as we have said, the increase is related more to the increase in numbers of drugs developed and consumed than to new and more harmful adverse effects.) But what people often don't understand is the reason that so many drugs have a toxic side to them. It is often said that a non-toxic drug is an ineffective one. This is because, at least with current methods of delivering the active ingredient, the drug will inevitably act on parts of the body other than the target cell or organ. If you take a drug by mouth, it will bathe every cell on the way down the digestive tract, and then, after being absorbed into the blood stream, it will bathe every cell in the body. Similarly, drugs given by injection will travel directly in the blood stream all over the body. At the moment, there is no way to make sure that a pill for migraine goes only to the head and another pill for gout goes only to the foot. The effect of this limitation on targeting drugs is twofold—first, the drugs might have beneficial effects on the target but inadvertently harmful effects on some of the other systems or organs and second, because any drug is diluted by the total volume of blood in the body, the patient has to take a much higher dose than is really necessary so that there is enough left by the time the diluted drug reaches the target. On its way, that higher dose may also exert harmful effects.

Pharmaceutical companies are beavering away at devising new methods of getting the molecules to exactly the place they are needed and nowhere else, but at the moment the vast majority of conventional remedies, and indeed unconventional remedies, that are taken by mouth or injection travel indiscriminately wherever they like.

But we have to accept that the absence of toxicity is a major attraction of most complementary medicines. And, as we've said, this is even more likely to be true with those remedies that are without efficacy against the disease. It may be the case that laetrile (or Essiac) are inactive against cancer, for example, but on the other hand they have far less toxicity than standard anti-cancer chemotherapy. In those situations where conventional chemotherapy for advanced cancer is of marginal benefit (and there are quite a few) the fact that complementary medicines have no side effects may be an important attraction.

Belief in treatment

Another feature that seems to be common to most complementary practitioners—and sometimes lacking in conventional doctors—is an unshakable faith in the efficacy of the treatment.

There are many contributory causes of this. First, by and large complementary practitioners move into their field by choice and with great conviction. Some have been given complementary medicines when they themselves were sick and they experienced improvements, some have seen patients who showed dramatic responses and some have spent a long time pondering and have been led to complementary medicine by an ever-deepening curiosity. Many complementary practitioners regard themselves as fundamentally sceptical but feel that they have been won over by the weight of evidence of cases and personal experience. Complementary practitioners are also quite likely to be practising exactly as they wish. Since there are many different variations of complementary medicine, there is a good chance of a new complementary practitioner specializing and finding some variation or combination of complementary medicines that he or she can become a local expert in.

This contrasts sharply with much of conventional medicine—particularly academic medicine—where only the brightest students follow their chosen career, and many doctors have to temper their ambition with an acknowledgement of what is feasible and politically practicable. In the past few years, the pressure on conventional doctors has risen. The career demands hard work, long hours, research (incurring the pressure to publish) and political savvy. Doctors (particularly junior doctors in hospitals) are quite often tired and harried—and are often most tired and most harried during patients' acute crises when patients and relatives are very sensitive to the doctor's personal style. Added to that, doctors have an obligation to be honest about their treatments and therefore have to explain when the treatment is likely to work and when it isn't. This truthfulness—demanded by law and by ethics—is often interpreted as lack of faith in the treatment. Clearly if the conventional doctor appears hassled, short of time and ambivalent about the therapy (as regards the statistics of success) the complementary practitioner who has total confidence in his or her therapy and is at ease and unhurried will present a more charismatic figure.

Local reputation

We often make some of our most important decisions for the most trivial reasons. We buy a house because the vendor had a vase full of flowers on the table (or was cleverly baking bread when we arrived), we marry someone because of an appealing smile (and quite often divorce him or her despite the same smile) and we buy cars in response to the most extraordinary appeals to our vanity and perceptions of social status and sexual functioning. Our attitudes in illness often contain the same elements—and one of the most powerful reasons for using a remedy or a form of medicine is that it worked for someone we know or have heard about. This seems to be a universal feaure of human behaviour (perhaps related to herd instincts and programming) and is just as true of doctors as of patients. A recent survey of doctors showed that although some of them read the medical literature and were impressed by the results of published studies, many were more influenced by a casual word from a respected colleague. It is easy to see that if the question is "Does this remedy *really* work?" the most intelligible answer is likely to be in the form of a personal anecdote. "It did wonders for Mrs. Brown's back" is a far more useful reply than "In seven clinical studies it produced an 8 per cent reduction in the Melzack pain index compared to placebo." We are deceived by the answer to the wrong question. We should be impressed not by the fact that Mrs. Brown got better *after* being treated, but by the fact that she got better *because* she was treated with homeopathic sepia. The first is a statement about chronology; the second about therapeutics.

It's because of the power of local reputation based on anecdotes that we have to investigate stories of miraculous recoveries so carefully—as we shall be doing in Chapter 7.

MINUSES OF CONVENTIONAL MEDICINE

So far then, we have seen most of the attractions of complementary medicine and seen some of the drawbacks of conventional medicine. This may be a useful point at which to summarize those features of the conventional consultation that cause most dissatisfaction.

Poor "people-doctoring"

Something has been lost from much of contemporary conventional medicine—a group of skills that we recognize as "good people-doctoring." We have detailed some of those features above (particularly aspects of support, personal involvement, caring, providing hope, giving listening time and acceptance). In some respects, these skills are part of the magic that should make up every consultation and with which conventional doctors seem somehow to have lost touch.

In fact, many of these skills—although natural to most complementary practitioners—can be taught to conventional doctors. In some universities, there are specialized teaching courses, which are sometimes called "The Science of the Art of Medicine"—a neat way of reminding students that even arts can be taught (to a certain extent).

However, in considering the loss of these personal "good doctor" skills, and to some extent in defence of the way conventional practice has evolved, we should be aware of the historical perspective.

As we discussed in Chapter 4, advances in drug therapy were few and far between until the 1930s. It has been suggested that at the turn of the century 96 per cent of the drugs in the pharmacopoeia were ineffective and were, in reality, placebos and nostrums. Most of the major conditions affecting patients—and particularly children—were infections. In dealing with a patient suffering from a major infection (whether it was acute, like pneumonia, or chronic, like TB), a doctor had to provide a great deal of support and empathy—there was little else to offer. It was hard work. Supporting a patient through a crisis of pneumonia or supporting the family if the patient died required a great deal of time and energy—family doctors after a round of house calls would feel totally drained. When effective drugs—particularly antibiotics—became available, the nature of many illnesses changed dramatically for patient and doctor. A prescription for a week's supply of antibiotics required much less from the doctor, and instead of repeated visits to suffering patients or grieving families, the doctor might make one or two follow-up visits or even have the recovered patient come to the office. Obviously, the requirement for support—part of the magic—decreased when effective drugs reached the market. It is no surprise that students in training during and after this period set much less store on their support skills—the pills seemed to be curing the ills.

Hence the beginning of the loss of the "magic" was not simply a matter of dazzling technology; it was also a diminution of the tragedy of irreversible illness. As we have seen already, the advances in the treatment of infectious diseases were not, unfortunately, followed by similar successes in all other human complaints, but the decline in "people-doctoring" had already begun—and has openly been in the process of reversal in the last decade or so.

The illusion of cure (a pill for every ill)

The idea that there is a pill for every ill brought with it a curious (and rather short-sighted) concept; if a patient had a problem for which no pill worked, doctors were trained to believe that perhaps the problem was not a "proper ill." Of course, once one has drawn the distinction between a disease and an illness this is not an issue. But 40 years ago, it was not accepted among the medical profession that illness without organic disease was common. This meant that doctors would constantly have to ignore very common symptoms—and the patients who brought them in—simply because there was "nothing in the book" that defined what the underlying disease was or how to treat it.

We now recognize that many patients have illnesses that are not caused by any organic disease, and this recognition will, in time, lead doctors away from the prescription pad, which may in turn decrease the incidence of iatrogenic side effects.

Losing touch

One other factor increased the loss of "people-doctoring": the use of technology in the process of diagnosis. Before X-rays and scans, doctors had to rely on their fingertips, eyes and ears to pick up diagnostic clues from the patient. Inevitably, this brought them into close physical contact with the patient and the act of touching—albeit for diagnostic purposes—changed the nature of the relationship. Even involuntarily, the touch had some magic in it.

As technology developed, physicians put greater and greater reliance on imaging techniques (X-rays and scans), objective blood tests, ECGs, EEGs and so on. This reliance was amplified considerably—particularly in the United States—as patients began to sue their doctors. Doctors whose only defence was "I heard crepitations at the lung bases" did poorly compared to doctors who had hard evidence—"The X-ray showed congestive cardiac failure, as you can see here."

This "distancing" meant that the doctors literally lost touch. Not only did they touch their patients less during diagnosis; they forgot how to use touch for support and as a symbol of empathy. The CT scanner is infinitely more sensitive to the presence of a cyst or a tumour than the doctor's finger, but unfortunately we have not yet built the scanner that is sensitive to the patient's feelings as well.

This chapter has been looking at the reasons for patients' migration from conventional medicine; hence, it has dealt only with the positive features of complementary medicine and the negative attributes of conventional doctors. This, however, is the perceived state of things in the eyes of those patients who are making that move. Perhaps we can summarize it—rather starkly—in the following table:

QUALITY	CONVENTIONAL DOCTOR	COMPLEMENTARY PRACTITIONER
Time	Usually rushed; average six minutes per patient	Unrushed; average 90 minutes for first consultation, 20 per follow-up
Setting	Usually depersonalized and institutionalized	Considerable effort made at patient's comfort and personalization
Continuity of care	Patient likely to see different person on follow-up visits	Patient usually sees same person
Symptom handling	Doctor trained to interpret patient's symptoms in light of knowledge of underlying disease. May "disbelieve" or contradict patient's view.	Accepts patient's symptoms at face value
Emotional handling	Empathic abilities are often poor	Empathic abilities are often central to practitioner's skill
Dealing with patient's personality	Doctor tries to compensate for or minimalize personal idiosyncrasies of patient	Practitioner regards patient's personal features as central to the illness and its treatment

QUALITY	CONVENTIONAL DOCTOR	COMPLEMENTARY PRACTITIONER
Dealing with social context	Variable. Importance of social context may be ignored or underestimated	Social context regarded as central to understanding of illness
Appearance of certainty	May appear uncertain; may be obliged to express both sides of a controversy	Usually certain and confident
Ability at giving clear prognosis	Obliged to be statistically accurate; answers may not seem clear or intelligible	Usually gives clear optimistic prognosis
Ability to give hope	Variable; usually not a major component of the relationship	Usually a major part of the relationship

7. ALTERNATIVE EXPLANATIONS OF THE INEXPLICABLE

> *"...if I told you I keep a goat in the backyard of my house in Florida,*
> *and if you happened to have a man nearby, you might*
> *ask him to look over my garden fence, when he'd say*
> *'That man keeps a goat.' But what would you do if I said,*
> *'I keep a unicorn in my backyard'?"*
> JAMES RANDI, *NATURE*, 1988, 334:287-290

> *No testimony is sufficient to establish a miracle*
> *unless the testimony be of such a kind that its falsehood would be more*
> *miraculous than the fact which it endeavours to establish.*
> DAVID HUME (1711-1776)

Nothing makes as compelling a story as somebody's amazing recovery from an awful disease against all the odds. It is powerful stuff. Think of the impact of a photograph of, say, a 60-year-old man at his granddaughter's second birthday party, when he had been told by his doctors that he would not survive to see her born. Or a newspaper photograph of a young child in a playground with a caption headed "Welcome Home Louisa" and explaining that her doctors had given up all hope, but with some locally raised funds she was taken to a special clinic in Mexico or Athens or Switzerland, and now here she is back home playing with her friends. Whether the story is headlined "Miracle Cure," "Back from the Brink Baby" or "Snatched from the Jaws of Death," eye-catchers like these have a tremendous impact on our thoughts about diseases and in particular about the treatment (conventional or complementary) that was used.

These stories appeal to the romance of an identifiable human struggle and the victory of spirit. They also are much easier to understand and absorb than dry medical facts. An article in a medical journal, for example, might show that bypass graft surgery extends the survival of patients with severe coronary-artery disease by approximately 15 per cent at six years compared to medical therapy alone. That information will mean almost nothing to most members of the public (and to some doctors, as well). However, the meaning becomes instantly clear when one sees the photograph of that 60-year-old man who was told he would be dead before his granddaughter was born. The statistics seem mundane; the personal example seems miraculous.

Because of the impact of dramatic "cures" on people's assessment of the therapy that led to it, it is important to find the real facts behind the story. This becomes even more important when you think about how such stories bolster the reputation of a clinic or treatment; even one apparent miracle per year with a particular form of treatment is quite enough to get droves of potential patients flying in from halfway across the world. So in this chapter, we will look at some of these events and in particular those recoveries that were unexpected or very surprising: the miracle or near-miracle cures. We shall ask an awkward question: Is the outcome a real miracle, or is there some other and less extraordinary explanation for what has happened?

In conventional medicine, a single unexpected response to a treatment will usually prompt the doctor in charge to publish a brief account in a professional journal—a case report. The case report, if it is thought to be sufficiently valuable, will be followed by a formal trial of the treatment in perhaps a handful of patients with the same disease. If those results show any responses, then a formal trial will be carried out to evaluate the therapy. In that way, the efficacy of the treatment is (or should be) tested and either confirmed or refuted. There are many examples of apparently dramatic responses to treatment that were later tested in formal trials, were shown to be ineffective and are no longer used.

By and large, this validation or confirmation process does not happen in complementary medicine. Case reports (until recently) would rarely be followed by formal trials of the treatment, even when the disease is common and a trial would be relatively easy to organize. Furthermore, published case reports in complementary medicine often have less stringent criteria for the diagnosis. In conventional medical journals, it would be usual to have important or crucial X-rays, scans or biopsy specimens re-examined by an independent expert in order to confirm that they show what they are supposed to show. Such double-checking is commonly absent from complementary medicine case reports.

NATURAL HISTORY OF THE DISEASE

Peter Morse is a man in his mid-twenties who developed a sudden pain behind his right eye. It came on suddenly while he was in a cinema, almost instantly he noticed that the movie appeared somewhat blurred when he shut his left eye and looked through his right eye only. The following day the ache behind the eye had not changed, and the vision in that eye was still blurred. He went to see a neurologist, who dismayed him when he told him that he had an inflammation of the nerve behind the eye and that it had a chance of progressing to multiple sclerosis. He immediately sought a herbalist, who started him on a variety of herbal remedies. Within two or three weeks, the pain and the blurring of vision had gone away. There have been no symptoms since that time, and Peter is convinced that the herbal remedies have cured him.

A story like this really does sound like a miracle. A hospital specialist said Peter had multiple sclerosis and the herbalist cured him. How could anyone doubt the miraculous power of the treatment? In fact, the answer may lie in acquiring a greater understanding of the problem that produced the symptoms and what happens as time goes on. In medical parlance, the way a disease progresses if it is not treated at all is called "the natural history" of the disease (as in "the natural history of a head cold is complete recovery in five to ten days").

So before anyone accepts any claims about the treatment of a disease, therefore, it is essential to find out more about what would have happened if no treatment had been used.

Self-limiting disease

Peter's initial problem in the eye was a condition called optic neuritis. It is true that in men, optic neuritis can be the first symptom of multiple sclerosis and approximately 30 per cent of males with optic neuritis will eventually develop multiple sclerosis. But for 70 per cent of patients, the episode of optic neuritis is all that ever happens. And even more important, in approximately 100 per cent of cases, the optic neuritis itself settles down in a few weeks. In other words, in all cases, optic neuritis is a self-limiting condition—its natural history is disappearance of the symptoms. Peter's problems would have disappeared even if he had not had any treatment at all. It is still possible (approximately a year after the neuritis) that he may develop other symptoms of multiple sclerosis, but the chance of that happening is 30 per cent. Either way, there is no connection between the herbal treatment and the fact that Peter's eye no longer troubles him.

This is one way in which a straightforward medical event can be interpreted as a miracle, when in fact nothing unusual actually happened.

The way in which a healer gains credit for giving any form of therapy at a time of natural recovery has been known for centuries. It was neatly and satirically expressed by John Earle (1601–1665) in his *Microcosmographie* when he wrote about the contemporary "meer dull physician" and said, "Though he be but an innocent bystander at some desperate recovery, yet he shall be blamed for it."

Fluctuations in disease

Brian Ledger had suffered from recurrent ulcers of the mouth and throat intermittently since he was 17 years old. Forty years later, having used homeopathic remedies for the last 12 years, he had experienced a dramatic change in his condition brought about, he believed, by the homeopathy. He has now been ulcer-free for several years.

However, the details of his story were quite important. When the ulcers of his mouth and throat began at age 17, they would last two or three weeks at a time and occurred every three or four months until he was 24. Then they disappeared for a period of four or five years, during which time he took no medicines. After that remission period, the ulcers returned with the same frequency and duration until, at the age of 45 (28 years after the start of the ulcer problem), he went to see a homeopath. He started taking the prescribed homeopathic medications for a few days at the onset of each attack of ulcers and noted that the attacks seemed to trouble him less. However, they still lasted as long and came as frequently for the first few years and then gradually decreased in severity and appeared at lengthened intervals until he was 54 years old, when they stopped altogether. By that time he had been taking the homeopathic remedy (intermittently with each attack) for a total of nine years. At the time of our interview, he had been almost totally ulcer-free for three years, during which time he had taken homeopathic tablets for a total of about ten days, whenever his throat felt a little sore.

Brian feels his situation is extremely unusual. He has never heard of anyone else with recurrent ulcers in the mouth and throat, and he is keen to publicize his case so that anyone else who has the problem can be told about homeopathic remedies to obtain relief.

Dr. Bill Tyldesly is the specialist in oral medicine at Brian's local dental hospital. The clinic at that hospital sees 3000 patients a year, of whom 16 per cent have recurrent mouth ulcers. It is the single commonest reason for a patient to see a specialist in oral medicine. There are three categories of recurrent oral ulcers: minor, major and herpetiform. The minor type of mouth ulcer does not cause major tissue damage to the soft palate or other major structures and typically lasts two to three weeks, recurring every three to four months; dozens of patients have had the problem longer than 20 years. Brian's story is typical of many patients in the commonest category of recurrent ulcers—the minor kind (although clearly the ulcers do not *feel* minor to the patients at the time). Of those patients troubled by minor mouth ulcers for more than 20 years, in many cases the condition will fluctuate for some years and then disappear completely. One of Dr. Tyldesly's recent patients was a woman who had had oral ulcers for 34 years and had been ulcer-free for just under three years.

So Brian's story is actually not particularly unusual for the natural history of recurrent mouth and throat ulcers, and his ulcers might easily have cleared up of their own accord (although it is still possible that they might recur in a few years). If this waxing-and-waning story is so common and is so commonly followed by total disappearance of the ulcers in so many cases, how can it be proven that in one case only, it was the homeopathy that caused the remission? The answer is: It can't. The improvement could simply be the natural course of events—and in Brian's case this is even more likely since he had already experienced a four- or five-year period of ulcer-free remission. Brian's history was rare and unusual to him but quite common to the specialists.

Mouth and throat ulcers of the minor category are very troublesome to the patient, but are not (medically speaking) a major illness, and they are certainly never life-threatening. So perhaps a fluctuating course and later disappearance of the problem might not be all that surprising. However, when the diagnosis is advanced cancer, most people think that the patient will deteriorate and die quickly—hence, any recovery without conventional therapy is often thought to be something of a miracle.

Audrey Parcell is a woman in her sixties who took the mistletoe extract iscadore and homeopathic remedies after doctors diagnosed a tumour in her abdomen.

Late in 1986, Audrey began to feel generally unwell and to lose her appetite. After some weeks, she began to have episodes of very severe abdominal pain. Her doctor examined her and found a large mass in the abdomen. After scans and X-rays, a needle aspirate was performed (that is, a sample of cells from the tumour was sucked out through a thin needle). The results of the aspirate showed that the mass was a lymphoma (a cancer of the lymph cells) of low-grade aggressiveness. The prognosis was portrayed to Audrey as quite gloomy (one doctor said, "You're so young...") but she did not want to try chemotherapy or radiotherapy. Instead, she saw a physician at the local Homeopathic Hospital and also went to the Bristol Cancer Help Centre. She started receiving regular injections of iscadore, took other oral homeopathic medicines and practised visualization techniques. She began to feel better in a few weeks, and within a few months the abdominal pain had disappeared and her appetite and weight recovered. She remains completely well now, and the latest ultrasound shows that the tumour in her abdomen is smaller (but still present).

Is this as extraordinary as it seems? One possibility might be misdiagnosis—Audrey was cured of a disease she didn't have. We took the specimens from the needle aspirate to a pathologist specializing in cancer and lymphoma in order to ensure that there was no mistake in the diagnosis. The review showed that the initial diagnosis was quite correct: the mass was almost certainly a low-grade lymphoma.

If the *diagnosis* was correct, was the *prognosis*—the doctor's estimate of how the patient might progress? The natural history of low-grade lymphomas holds the key to understanding what might have gone on in this case. Low-grade lymphomas are not only slow-growing tumours that may take many years to cause trouble, but in a high proportion of cases, the tumours fluctuate, getting bigger and smaller without any treatment at all; for example, a low-grade lymphoma may produce lumps under the patient's armpit or in the neck. The lumps may grow to several inches across and then disappear over a period of several months without any treatment. In a small number of cases, all visible masses may disappear totally for periods of up to a few years.

The natural history of this type of lymphoma almost always seems odd to the patient who hears the word "cancer" and expects rapid progression of a lethal disease. In Audrey's case, a conventional cancer specialist would have recommended treatment while she was feeling ill with the loss of weight and abdominal pain. But even without treatment, there was perhaps a one-in-ten chance that there would have been improvement in her symptoms (and the mass in her abdomen).

This understanding of the natural history of the tumour may be very disquieting for the patient, and particularly for those who feel that their regime (be it diet, iscadore or anything else) has caused the improvement. Patients who believe they have been cured miraculously can be unimpressed by an explanation of the natural history of the disease and feel far more comfortable believing that the treatment has cured them.

Premature follow-up

In Tijuana, Mexico, a woman in her early forties comes to a clinic to receive laetrile and coffee enemas for her cancer. She is extremely optimistic that the complementary medicine will work in her case. She had breast cancer diagnosed approximately six months previously. The tumour was relatively small (about two centimetres) and the surgeon had told her that one lymph node in the armpit had cancer in it. As is routine in this situation, the surgeon had referred the patient to a medical oncologist (cancer specialist) who had given the patient six courses of chemotherapy to try to prevent any recurrence of the cancer. After the chemotherapy, she had booked the trip to Tijuana.

This particular patient was included in the statistics of the Tijuana clinic and was listed as a patient who had shown response to laetrile in that she now had no evidence of cancer. However that wasn't really the truth of the matter.

A patient with a small cancer of the breast and one lymph node involved has approximately an 87 per cent chance of living for five years. In other words, in only 13 per cent of cases would a patient like this woman die of her disease within five years. The chance of the cancer coming back in a few months (that is, when she was at the Tijuana clinic) would be nearly zero. Therefore the claim that the patient had no evidence of cancer *because of* the laetrile was simply wrong. The patient was free of disease because she had a relatively good prognosis based on her small tumour—added to which she had already received appropriate conventional therapy that had improved her chances even further.

One problem in interpreting such stories is that the triumphal return of a patient from a foreign clinic is big news; if the patient later dies, that is not big news and sometimes isn't even reported in the popular media.

A typical front-page story in this category was that of a lovely young girl, "Missy" Duvall, who was taken by her parents to Athens (actually to Dr Alivizatos, whose career we mentioned in Chapter 5) after her doctors in Toronto told her there was nothing more that they could do to treat her neuroblastoma (a rare cancer of childhood). Missy and her family went to the Alivizatos clinic and Missy was given the doctor's complete treatment with secret serums and diets. Missy returned to Toronto and was the subject of many stories in the media. Unfortunately, she began to deteriorate and died several months after her return from Athens. Her death was reported in the papers but (obviously) with much less space devoted to it. Even fairly diligent readers of the newspapers may still have the impression that Missy Duvall was the "kid who was saved by that doctor in Athens."

One of the most famous of all these cases was the tragic death of the actor Steve McQueen from a mesothelioma (asbestos-induced cancer of the lining of the chest) in 1980. Steve McQueen was diagnosed as having a mesothelioma in December 1979 and chemotherapy was recommended. He declined (which in view of the poor success rate with conventional chemotherapy was probably a sound decision) and went to the Plaza Santa Maria clinic in Mexico. He received a large number of complementary medicine therapies (chosen from a repertoire including coffee enemas, rectal enzyme implants, aloe vera, Bach flower remedies, pancreatic enzyme tablets, reflexology and castor oil hot packs). According to the medical team there, these treatments produced "tremendous clinical biochemical improvement" with some of the biochemical markers of cancer in his blood becoming negative. The team then decided to operate on McQueen to remove tumours that they felt had shrunk. He survived the five-hour operation but died of heart failure 14 hours later on November 7. McQueen's death was made even more tragic by the fact that he believed himself to have been cured. On October 6, he had announced that "Mexico is showing the world this new way of fighting cancer through nonspecific metabolic therapy. Congratulations and thank you for helping to save my life." His statement was emotional and heartfelt. Very few people would have had the nerve to disagree with any statement coming from a man as adored and revered as McQueen was, particularly a statement of such courage and optimism. Despite the sincere hopes of the patient, his doctors and his audience, unfortunately Steve McQueen wasn't cured and he died a short time later. Yet such is the power of a premature statement or promise of cure, that even today many people believe Steve McQueen was almost cured at the Mexican clinic and died as a result of mischance. The widespread survival of that belief is a demonstration of the power and popularity of premature claims.

Spontaneous regressions

The phrase spontaneous regression really means "This disease almost always gets worse, but on this occasion it went away and nobody knows why." Certain criteria have to be met before a patient's improvement can be accepted as a true spontaneous regression. The disease has to be proven by biopsy; otherwise the diagnosis might be wrong. (Several cases of miracle cures of cancer of the pancreas later turned out to be misdiagnosis and were actually chronic pancreatitis, which very often gets better by itself.) When the diagnosis is correct, the disease must be seen to be progressing at the time of stopping all known active treatment. A spontaneous regression is then defined as improvement in all areas of disease and the patient's return to health. The regression is termed complete if the disease has disappeared totally, and partial if it has improved but not disappeared altogether. The phrase is most commonly used about cancers, but it can apply to any disease that is universally progressive or irreversible.

While investigating reports of unusual regressions, we came across the story of Tom Wolland, which was extraordinary in almost every aspect.

> Tom was two and a half years old when he suddenly developed weakness in his right leg and general unsteadiness, which became dramatically worse over a few days until he was scarcely able to walk or stand.

His concerned parents took him to the local neurosurgeon, who ordered a CT scan. The scan showed a large cyst with some tumour in the wall. The cyst was so large that it was compressing the back part of Tom's brain, causing the paralysis and unsteadiness. It would have been technically impossible to perform a biopsy or remove the cystic tumour without maiming or killing Tom. The neurosurgeon told Tom's parents that the probable diagnosis was a malignant brain tumour called an astrocytoma and that the prognosis was bleak. He recommended radiotherapy.

Tom's parents were great believers in complementary medicine and immediately started Tom on a diet of carp soup and burdock. They also instigated regular prayers (they are both practising Buddhists) and took Tom to a homeopathic doctor. Tom seemed to benefit from none of these treatments but continued to deteriorate steadily, becoming more and more disabled and less and less active. He was given one single dose of radiotherapy a few weeks after diagnosis but was simply unable to tolerate the immobilization required, so it was abandoned.

About three months after the diagnosis when Tom was still deteriorating progressively, an extraordinary event occurred that seemed to change everything. While the family was visiting some friends, Tom picked up a small rubber ball and got it jammed in his mouth. It choked him and he fell to the ground spluttering and choking. He quickly went blue and then black and stopped breathing. His parents started a series of Buddhist chants but one of their friends was more active and struggled with the ball. After a few minutes, he managed to dislodge it. Tom did not start to breathe after the ball was removed, but the same friend did some mouth-to-mouth resuscitation and Tom revived.

Tom's parents are convinced that his recovery began on that day. From that moment on, he slowly regained his mental vigour and the use of his right arm and leg, and now at the age of six, he is virtually a normal child. His latest CT scan shows that the cyst is considerably smaller and, as before, does not show any distinct mass or lump of tumour. His parents do not know exactly what it was that made him better, but they think it was mostly due to the various complementary medicines that Tom had been taking—and that the choking episode helped him turn the corner in some way.

This story is an extraordinary one, but Tom's parents are almost certainly correct about their second conclusion—attributing the start of the recovery to the choking episode. Although there is no biopsy evidence, the cyst originally seen in the back part of Tom's brain of the scan was probably part of a brain tumour called an astrocytoma, just as Tom's doctors suspected. Astrocytomas in children often contain fluid-filled spaces, in other words, cysts, so the probable diagnosis fits the data quite well. In adults this type of cancer is usually relative fast-growing and is difficult to treat, but in children these tumours are much more variable and unpredictable. In fact, astrocytomas in children can be quite slow-growing and can shrink or even disappear spontaneously. On average, a paediatric neurologist will see one or two spontaneous regressions of childhood astrocytomas in about 20 years of specialist practice.

So in Tom's case, it was possible that the original cyst was part of an astrocytoma that grew steadily over several months—but how did it happen that Tom suddenly seemed to start improving after the choking episode? One thing that is very likely to help a cyst to rupture is increased pressure inside the head, and one of the commonest ways in which the pressure inside the head can be raised—as you might have guessed—is by coughing and spluttering. The attempt to breathe out when the airway is closed (or in Tom's case, when the mouth is sealed with a rubber ball) is called the Valsalva manouevre (weightlifters do it while lifting, and most of us do it when we vomit or strain for any reason), and it can raise the intracranial pressure to dramatically high levels. In Tom's case, this rise in pressure followed by the sharp decrease in pressure as he became unconscious almost certainly caused the rupture of the big cyst at the back of his brain and that rupture was followed by his gradual recovery. Although that may seem somewhat strange at first, it is well-known that cysts inside the brain are quite liable to rupture—either spontaneously[1] or after injury to the head[2] (which might be comparable to Tom's situation).

Of course, this explanation—however plausible—can never be proven since it was not possible to do a biopsy on the original tumour.

So the true diagnosis and the real sequence of events in Tom's case will never be known, but the same is also true of all the other possible explanations. Furthermore, the explanations involving the other treatments that Tom had been given were also badly flawed. He had already been on the carp soup and burdock for over three months and had been taking homeopathic remedies for the same amount of time, during which period he had deteriorated continuously. The same was true of all the other various recipes and herbs, as well as the prayers. The radiotherapy was given at one-eighth of its intended dose and was given months before the recovery. The only thing that was definitely associated with the turn-around in Tom's condition—according to his parents—was the choking episode. The rupture of a cyst inside an astrocytoma fits the data perfectly. Certainly it's a very unusual situation, but it is quite compatible with what we know about brain cancer in children and with what we know of human physiology and increased intracranial pressure. Not that it would be recommended to any other patient, but choking almost to death probably saved Tom's life.

This is a very dramatic and highly unusual example of a spontaneous regression (or at least a natural regression, if one considers that swallowing a ball is not really a spontaneous event). However, the great Canadian pathologist William Boyd collected a series of over 200 stories of spontaneous remissions for which there is faultless documentation over a period of 80 years.[3]

A woman of 23 went to her doctor with a mole that was growing on her right foot. The mole had developed black satellite nodules around it, and the doctor correctly diagnosed a rare and aggressive skin cancer called malignant melanoma. It was nearly two inches in diameter and was removed surgically. The specimen was confirmed as a melanoma. It has often been suggested that malignant melanoma gets worse if the patient becomes pregnant and because of this, the patient was advised that she shouldn't become pregnant—but she did. In fact, she became pregnant less than six months after her operation, and secondaries from her malignant melanoma appeared very rapidly over her right leg and thigh. Even more ominously, her liver began to enlarge, and it was generally considered that the outlook was hopeless. Nevertheless, without any treatment at all, her liver began to shrink three months after her first baby was born. She became pregnant again and after the second pregnancy the skin secondaries began to get smaller, disappearing completely after her third child. Biopsies of the faded lesions confirmed that there was now no evidence of active cancer at that site. She actually went on to have two more healthy children (making five in all since the diagnosis of the melanoma) and remained completely well until nearly ten years after the initial diagnosis. At that time, she suddenly developed secondaries of melanoma in many areas of her body and died within six months.

It's easy to see with a case like this how the phenomenon of spontaneous regression, if it occurs at the time the patient is taking some treatment—alternative or conventional—could give the overwhelming impression that the treatment is responsible for the patient's improvement. It highlights one of the dangers of paying too much attention to individual cases.

Another major survey of cases of spontaneous regression looked at over 1000 reported cases. Of that number, only 130 cases actually had enough documentation to prove the diagnosis and the regression.[4] And from that set of cases, two very significant facts emerged. The first one is that spontaneous regressions occur (approximately) once in every 100,000 cases of cancer. Hence in a cancer centre that sees, let's say, 5000 new patients a year, a spontaneous regression would be seen every 20 years.

The second point is even more surprising. The frequency with which spontaneous regressions occur depends on the type of cancer. Although the occasional spontaneous regression is seen in almost every type of cancer known, over half of the regressions occur in four types of cancer. They are neuroblastoma (a tumour of primitive nerve cells usually occurring in young children), malignant melanoma (the black mole cancer of the skin mentioned above), choriocarcinoma (cancer of the placenta) and renal cell carcinoma (cancer of the kidney).

It's important to note that spontaneous regressions are well-documented (and every centre of pilgrimage ought to be reporting at least one per 100,000 cases of cancer). Because of our inbuilt urge to make causal connections between contiguous events, even a single case of spontaneous regression can be easily accepted quickly and widely as evidence that the treatment given at the time really worked.

MISINTERPRETATION

There are several different ways in which information can be mishandled and can give the wrong impression to the patient—or doctor. Sometimes a situation that is not clear and is full of "ifs," "buts" and "maybes" is explained or understood poorly. As a result, the patient may have a view of the disease or the prognosis that is a long way from the medical facts. Then, again, sometimes the patient understands the information perfectly well but has been given the wrong information in the first place.

MISINTERPRETATION OF INFORMATION

Jim Collins is someone whose experience with cancer could be seen as an illustration of the effects of spiritual healing. A lump appeared on his left thigh; it grew rapidly and was soon the size of an orange. At the local hospital, a biopsy was done, which showed that the mass was a liposarcoma, a rare and aggressive form of cancer. Obviously the diagnosis was a major shock to Jim, but there was worse to come. As part of the routine work-up, Jim had a CT scan of his lungs to see if there were any secondaries from the liposarcoma. Sadly, there were half a dozen small nodules seen at the base of the left lung and around the back of both the left and right lungs. The doctors told Jim about the secondaries. Jim, by coincidence, had recently completed a project in cancer statistics and realized that his chance of surviving with secondaries in his lungs from a sarcoma was less than 5 per cent. The situation looked gloomy. Jim, however, was determined not to give in and undertook a major program of reorganizing his life and personality. He prayed a great deal, rethought his personal priorities in his life and started a major program of physical fitness (though he had always been reasonably fit and active).

Jim was referred to a radiotherapy centre for local treatment to his thigh to make sure that, at the very least, the cancer did not recur at the local site. His doctors repeated the CT scan of his lungs three months after the first one to see how fast the secondaries were growing. At the second scan, the nodules were exactly the same size. At the third scan six months later, and the fourth scan a year later, the nodules were also absolutely static. By this time, Jim was so fit that he was able to run up the tallest mountain in Wales—a major achievement measured on any scale.

Such a detailed and dramatic account suggests that something unusual occurred to prevent Jim's decline and help him turn the corner. Although Jim never overtly claimed that his regime of prayer and exercise was directly responsible for the state of his cancer, he clearly believes that something of a miracle had happened—but had it?

Jim's story is, surprisingly, not a rare one. The problem is that as CT scans have become more and more routine, doctors are seeing abnormalities that are quite common and are insignificant. When the doctors reviewed Jim's first CT scans and compared them with the second set three months later, it became clear that there was another far more likely explanation of the small nodules—benign scarring, probably a result of asbestos exposure many years previously. In fact, Jim had never had secondaries in his lungs, but with the discovery of the aggressive tumour in his thigh, those nodules in the lungs had been (appropriately) interpreted as secondaries, since, on balance, this was the most likely (and important) explanation in a man with an aggressive cancer in his thigh. Although benign lung nodules are actually very common, the doctors looking after Jim felt that it was far more important to take a very cautious—and therefore pessimistic—view to start with. In that way, if the nodules turned out later to be benign, all concerned would be delighted. On the other hand, if the doctors had assumed the nodules to be innocent but they had later turned out to be malignant, the effect on Jim would have been catastrophic.

Jim himself was informed about the revised diagnosis at the three-month stage and naturally was overjoyed (as, by the way, were all his doctors). It is easy to see how a misinterpretation like this could have been inflated into a major claim that diet, prayer, exercise and a change in attitude can change the course of cancer.

The fact of the matter is that medicine is not a precise science, although everyone (patients and doctors alike) wishes it were. CT scans are a good example of this; sometimes the scan shows instantly what is wrong, sometimes it shows clearly that nothing is wrong, but quite often it shows some abnormalities that could be a sign of serious trouble or could be nothing to worry about at all. Nodules in the lungs are quite common findings in the normal population, but early secondaries from cancer can look exactly like them. The normal routine in that situation is, as happened in Jim's case, to repeat the scan a little later and see what has happened in the course of time (unless you can do an exploratory operation to find out—which, if the nodules are small or deep, is not recommended).

In medicine we often have to be content with less than a perfect answer. Sometimes, as in Jim's case, the doctors take the most pessimistic explanation because it is the most likely one and, in a few cases (such as Jim's), later revise the gloomy outlook into a brighter one. This is not a miracle—it's a revision.

Of course, to some people this will seem like needless hair-splitting. Whether Jim didn't have secondaries to start with or had them and they disappeared may not matter; he hasn't got them now and that's the important thing. And if there's a *possibility* that prayer helped, why search assiduously for other explanations? This raises a number of issues to do with alternative medicine as a whole, and we will explore them more fully later.

Wrong information

Sometimes, the patient is given wrong information by the healer, but understands it quite correctly. This may be a less common cause of misinterpretation but is often quite difficult to unravel. The following case is a typical example, observed during a morning in a London acupuncture clinic:

Denise Bray was diagnosed by the healer as having three major problems: a stuffed-up nose, a bladder infection and arthritis. Her story was taken by two trainee acupuncturists and then reviewed by the senior acupuncturist. The senior person explained that the patient had had arthritis for many years and had obtained much relief from her acupuncture. She had recently had an asthma attack for which she had been prescribed a steroid inhaler, which had produced improvement in the asthma. However, the senior acupuncturist said, the chi lines from the lungs are closely connected to the bladder and so it was no surprise that the patient immediately developed a bladder infection, which required more acupuncture. The condition had now been cleared up entirely by acupuncture.

To a medical observer, this explanation was astonishing. It is possible that symptoms such as pain and even the feeling of stuffiness in the nose could be improved by acupuncture. But it was difficult to imagine how acupuncture could possibly clear up an infection in the bladder. After all, bacteria causing damage in the wall of the bladder are separate living organisms; if acupuncture genuinely killed them, then the only way it could work was by affecting the immune system. The senior acupuncturist was quite certain that this is what had happened. Indeed, the patient confirmed that her bladder infection had gone away.

In fact, going over the story again with the patient, there was a much more prosaic explanation. Two weeks previously, Denise had awoken in the night to pass urine twice, which was unusual for her. The following night, she passed urine three times. On the third night, she passed urine twice again. It appeared that the urine did not sting, it did not smell peculiar, she did not pass urine more often than usual during the day and never had any urgency (a strong desire to pass urine). All these symptoms are cardinal features of a bladder infection—and this patient had had none of them. In other words, nothing in Denise's story suggested that she had had a bladder infection in the first place. One further question made the solution even clearer; she had had her urine tested by her family doctor before she came to the acupuncture centre and the doctor had told her that the urine test showed no infection at all.

Clearly then, although Denise had unexpectedly passed urine several times in each of three successive nights, she had never had a bladder infection. Yet her acupuncturists had told her that she had had an infection and felt that they had cured it with the acupuncture. Without a doctor asking some ordinary medical questions, Denise might well have believed that she had had an infection and that it had been cured by acupuncture. After all, this is what the acupuncturist told her, and the patient would have to be very confident of the signs and symptoms of bladder infection to argue with her healer.

Was this a miracle cure? Certainly the patient was delighted with the effects of the acupuncture, but she didn't call it a miracle. The acupuncturists spoke of it in even more matter-of-fact tones, as if everybody knew that acupuncture could cure bacterial infections. Only to a conventional doctor did this (at first) appear to be a miracle, in the sense that if it were true, it would have demanded a dramatic re-thinking of human pathology and physiology. In the event, there was no unicorn in the garden. If it was anything, it was a goat.

Heather Haynes went to register with a family doctor when she moved to a new neighbourhood. She had no recent health problems, but mentioned that a few years previously, at the age of 38, she had had a stroke affecting her left side. She told the family doctor that she had visited a herbalist at the time, and that with the herbal remedies she had been given, she had made a complete recovery.

A stroke at the age of 38 is very rare in women, and when it happens it is usually caused by problems with blood pressure or blood clotting. The family doctor thought this was very important and asked more questions. Heather had not had any problems relevant to a stroke before the incident and had had no problems since. In fact, she added, the stroke had been quite mild and affected only the left side of her face.

The doctor examined Heather carefully and found the answer. When he asked Heather to raise her eyebrows, she could raise only the right eyebrow fully; on the left side, the eyebrow lifted only slightly and she could not wrinkle her forehead properly on that side. All other muscles of the face were normal, but that weakness gave the doctor the answer. Heather had not had a stroke at all. She had had an inflammation of the facial nerve called a Bell's palsy.

The facial nerve is a long thin nerve that travels out into the facial muscles through a winding canal in the skull. It quite frequently becomes inflamed (often after a mild virus infection), and when it swells up it squashes itself and produces a paralysis of half the face. That paralysis includes the forehead on that side. If Heather had had a stroke (i.e., if the damage was not in the nerve but way above it in the brain itself), the forehead would not be paralyzed because it so happens that each side of the forehead muscles receives signals from each side of the brain. So if Heather had had a stroke in the right side of her brain, she would have lost the use of the left side of her lower face but her left forehead would have been normal. As it was, her left forehead was paralyzed, so the damage could not have been in the brain, but must have been in the nerve. A Bell's palsy in a 38-year-old woman is by no means rare, and recovery occurs in a few weeks (exactly as it had done in Heather's case).

This was a minor but important point of diagnosis, but it did mean that Heather was in no danger from a future stroke. It also meant that the herbalist could not legitimately claim that he had cured a stroke.

These cases pose a most important question—and one that has several possible answers. The question is: Does it matter? The answer depends on who is asking. If one sees this from the patient's viewpoint, of course it does not matter. One patient had some episodes of passing urine at night that had disappeared while she had her acupuncture; the other made a complete recovery from an apparent stroke. From their viewpoint, there were no problems: The treatments made them feel better. Any quibbles simply did not matter to them.

However, there are other viewpoints. The acupuncturists believed (and still do believe) that acupuncture is as good as antibiotics for some infections (for example, of the bladder). The herbalist believed that herbal remedies cure strokes. Do those beliefs matter? The answer is that they do matter if, believing those observations to be fact, the practitioners then suggest that acupuncture should be used with all patients with bladder infections or herbs for strokes. Some patients will have genuine bladder infections and will be given treatment that doesn't cure them, and some patients with a stroke won't be sent to their own doctors to have their blood pressure checked and future strokes prevented. From that point of view, it does matter. Although the patient's view may be an alternative to the scientist's view, there is no alternative to truth. Acupuncture does not cure bladder infections, but it does make patients feel better. Herbal remedies don't cure strokes, but Bell's palsies get better by themselves. And that distinction is important and does matter.

Perhaps on the wide scale of human illness, bladder infections and Bell's palsies are troublesome but not of major significance. However, the diagnosis of fatal and terminal illness is altogether a different matter, and anyone claiming that they are curing cancers, for example, will be raising the hopes of thousands of desperate and vulnerable people.

At the age of 58, a man suffered a sudden episode of transient confusion, followed by an inability to speak followed by a loss of consciousness and then a grand mal convulsive fit. He was admitted to hospital where his brain scan and skull X-ray were found to be normal, but there was an abnormal epileptic focus of electrical activity in his EEG. He made a complete recovery and was discharged from hospital on anticonvulsant drugs.

Three years later, the patient suffered a very sudden loss of awareness during a bus journey and missed his bus stop. He thought that he had dozed off but in the next 24 hours developed headaches followed quickly by clumsiness, inability to do simple tasks and then drowsiness. He was admitted to hospital on the third day of this illness when a CT scan showed a patch of something in the right frontal lobe surrounded by mushy swelling of the brain. The initial report suggested that it was a tumour. No biopsy was possible. The patient was started on steroids to reduce the swelling and made an excellent recovery. He left hospital on the eleventh day of his illness.

Three months after his second hospital admission, he was seen for the first time by a homeopathic physician. The patient was suffering from side effects of the steroids, which were being slowly reduced in dose. The homeopathic physician gave the patient various remedies, and the patient's recovery continued uninterrupted. Three years after the illness, a repeat CT scan shows only a few abnormalities in the area of the problem—notably some thinning of the brain substance.

The homeopathic physician published a report in a homeopathic journal as a case of space-occupying lesion (a lump), probably glioma (cancer of the brain), that had responded to homeopathic remedies.

If a proven brain cancer (glioma) was genuinely cured after the administering of homeopathic remedies, this would be a real unicorn in the garden. Moreover, even among unicorns, it would be a rarity since brain cancer is notoriously difficult to treat with *any* therapy and sometimes responds to only the highest doses of chemotherapy or radiotherapy. It is not an easily tameable tumour.

In fact, this patient almost certainly suffered from two strokes (one three years previously, and the second causing this illness) and never had a brain tumour of any description. Even on the patient's story alone, the occurrence of two very sudden episodes of brain disturbance is quite typical of the way strokes affect patients. They are actually called "strokes" precisely because of this sudden appearance. Patients can also recover completely from strokes in a short time (if the patient recovers in less than 24 hours, the stroke is a transient ischaemic attack or "mini-stroke"). By contrast, brain tumours usually cause symptoms to develop slowly over several weeks or several days at the least, although very occasionally there can be bleeding inside a tumour, which may make it appear to cause symptoms suddenly. However, given the fact that this patient had an episode three years previously from which he made a full recovery, the betting should be very heavily on this current problem being a stroke, not a cancer.

Most important, though, the CT scan shows something that could easily be a stroke. The scan shows a white lump about two centimetres across. It is white on the scan because some dye has been injected into the patient's veins, making the blood vessels look white. The lump is therefore full of blood. It could be a very vascular tumour, true, but it is quite typical of a stroke. It is surrounded by swelling, which is also quite typical of a stroke (although it often occurs around tumours as well). The patient made a quick recovery due to the swelling being diminished by steroids. Three years later, that area of the brain is slightly thinned, a typical finding after a stroke.

The history, the CT scan and the progress are all typical of stroke. Although the CT scan appearance was certainly compatible with brain cancer (and the X-ray physician who looked at it was not wrong if he or she had said, "It could be a tumour"), the appearance was also quite compatible with a stroke.

If it was a stroke, it was typical—it was the second one in this patient, he made a full recovery from both and everything fits perfectly. If it was a brain cancer, then it is the most unusual one ever recorded since it didn't behave like one to begin with, got better with steroids and then disappeared after three years of homeopathy.

How easy is it to get muddled between a tumour and a stroke? The answer is: very easy. Even with the results of a CT scan, it can quite often be very difficult to distinguish between the two. Most neurologists and neurosurgeons have had experience of at least three or four cases in which it was very difficult to tell whether the patient had a tumour or a stroke. In one case seen in Toronto,[5] the diagnosis of a stroke was made only when the patient had a biopsy. In other words, the appearance of the CT scan looked like a tumour to the radiologist, it looked like a tumour to the neurosurgeon and it behaved like a tumour with slowly increasing symptoms and progressive paralysis. The patient was taken to the operating room and a fine needle advanced carefully into the abnormal area of the brain to take a small specimen of what—everybody assumed—would turn out to be a tumour. The pathologist analyzed the specimen under the microscope and found there was no tumour at all—it was a stroke. Naturally the medical team was pleased for the patient, as was he when he came round from the anaesthetic, and his recovery after the operation was far better than it would have been if he'd had a tumour. It was almost miraculous, in fact.

This is not unique; mistaken diagnoses underlie quite a few apparently miraculous cures, particularly in patients who apparently have cancer.

From time to time, cases are reported of patients who showed all the signs of serious cancer in their bodies, of a type that doctors felt was untreatable, and who were therefore given palliative treatment and told that they had only a short time to live, after which they confounded the doctors and lived to a ripe old age. An interesting study was reported in the *British Medical Journal* in 1987[6]; it hints at the possibility that large numbers of such patients were given a mistaken diagnosis in the first place and had never had cancer. Two of the doctors who carried out the study worked in a hospice to which patients were referred for terminal care. Among the 1635 patients referred over a period, four turned out not to have the disease that had been diagnosed originally. One woman, for example, had had an abdominal operation, during the course of which her entire pancreas was found to be affected by cancer, which was infiltrating the surrounding structures. The disease was deemed inoperable and the diagnosis put in her notes. Four years later, she had multiple abdominal pains for which she required painkillers, and the hospital treating her then referred her to the hospice for terminal care. As one of the doctors reported, "She looked remarkably well for a woman with terminal pancreatic cancer." Eventually, on further investigation, it turned out that her pancreas was now perfectly normal and that she must have had pancreatitis, a non-cancerous inflammation of the pancreas that can be notoriously difficult to distinguish from cancer.

Another patient had a malignancy diagnosed on the basis of a sample of fluid from the lining of his lungs; it contained cells that looked cancerous. He was admitted to the hospice for terminal care and five months later, upon reinvestigation, he was found to be free of the disease. The doctors conclude that the original diagnosis was a misreading of the fluid sample and that there had never been cancer there at all. Three years later, the patient was robust, cheerful and maintaining a completely independent existence.

Extrapolated to the population of Britain, four in 1635 hospice admissions could mean that hundreds of patients each year were believed to recover mysteriously from fatal cancer that never existed. This research is relevant to our topic, of course, because if such patients had consulted an alternative therapist for treatment for the "disease" that conventional medicine had deemed incurable, it would have been very difficult not to ascribe the subsequent "recovery" to the effects of the alternative therapy.

Selective recall

Medicine, as we have said many times in this book, is an imprecise science. In fact, as we shall see in the next chapter, quite large chunks of it are not science at all. But there is one area in which most patients and family members want precise scientific answers from their doctors and have a tendency to endow whatever the doctor says with a scientific accuracy that simply doesn't exist. The area in question is the prognosis of the disease, and for the more serious diseases, the question that most people want answered is "How long have I got?"

The fact of the matter is that "How long have I got?" is a very difficult question to answer, and although conventional medicine is quite effective at providing predictions for groups (for example, distinguishing a high-risk group from a low-risk one), there is very little that is of real help when an individual patient asks a specific question of an individual doctor.

In some respects, this is simply an illustration of the large gap between general information and specific information; for example, if an airline loses luggage one time out of 10,000 (i.e., 0.01 per cent of the time), that doesn't help you very much if it happens to be your suitcase that they send to Dusseldorf while you fly to Los Angeles. For you—and your suitcase—that loss is not 0.01 per cent, it's 100 per cent. Statistics are, of course, very helpful *before* you decide which airline to use, but are not much help once you're committed. For instance, the fact that Volksluft Airlines loses luggage 0.0001 per cent of the time, whereas Fly By Night Airlines loses it 12 per cent of the time may help you decide which airline you will use. However, the statistics themselves are only of minor consolation if you happen to be the one victim of Volksluft's luggage-handling fallibility.

It is that gap—between the statistical and the personal—that angers and frustrates many patients. On some occasions, the anger and frustration are made worse by a doctor's poor communication skills. Sometimes the doctor is just a poor communicator, but quite often even a good communicator may be discomfited or even frightened and make things worse by trying to cover up any awkwardness with what he or she thinks is cool professional poise. It is quite common to hear of patients and families deeply upset and angered by discussions about prognoses with their doctors.

The desire to try to convey the whole picture makes things even worse for the doctors. Because they are usually trying to convey the idea of a range of prognoses (i.e., the possible outcomes for an entire group of patients with this particular condition), doctors are often perceived as hedging and trying to avoid telling the truth. The patient is quite likely to suspect that the doctor knows the exact answer but is unwilling or afraid to give it. Hence many patients seize on one aspect of the doctor's answer and hold on to it, believing it to be the genuine and accurate truth of the matter, which they have managed to ferret out of the doctor, despite his or her attempt to cover it up.

It is quite surprising how often this happens in clinical practice. Let's take as an example a condition such as oat-cell cancer of the lung. This is a condition that makes up about 20 per cent of all lung cancers. It is a fairly rapidly growing tumour and has a strong tendency to spread to distant parts of the body. Of any group of patients with oat-cell lung cancer, the average patient survival is about 14 to 16 months. Statistically, that means that of 100 patients, 50 will survive for less than that time, and 50 will live longer. In fact, approximately 15 per cent will still be alive at two years and 5 per cent will be alive at five years. That is quite a complicated situation for a doctor to explain to a patient; it is quite difficult to understand it as an intellectual exercise, but it is much more difficult when the listener is hearing information about his or her own life or death. Here is a typical example of how the conversation might go:

PT: So how long have I got?
DR: It's very difficult to say, Mr. Brown. The disease is quite serious and it's likely to advance in months rather than several years.

PT: You mean I might die in a few months?

DR: Well, I'm sorry to say that it's possible. Patients with this disease can live several years—a few patients may still be doing well after five years or more—but it's quite often a matter of many months or a small number of years rather than several years.

PT: But I've got my daughter's wedding in three months' time. Surely you can guarantee that I'll be OK for that.

DR: I wish I could guarantee it unconditionally. I must say it's quite likely that you'll be fine, but there is still a small chance that the disease might go very fast in your particular case.

PT: Are you saying I might not be around in three months?

DR: I'm only saying that that's a possibility. It's not a big chance that things would go that badly, but the chance exists. By and large, most patients live longer than that—and obviously we have every hope you will—but we can't guarantee it.

PT: I see.

Many patients will take all this to mean that the real prognosis is three months and that the doctor talked about some patients living five years only in order to make things sound better than they are. Therefore, when they tell anyone else about the conversation, they are quite likely to say (and believe), "The doctor's given me three months."

This may make a considerable difference if the patient then goes to another doctor or healer and tries some new treatment. For instance, at one clinic in California, the medical staff actually write down what the patient says about the prognosis when the patient arrives. If the patient says, "The doctor gave me three months," that is recorded as the real prognosis, and it is not checked or verified with the original doctor or in any other way. If the patient then survives twice as long—six months in this case—the clinic regards that as a success for its treatment and says so in its annual analysis. This particular approach is clearly not based on reliable and verified data, and many people would feel that this method of claiming success is verging on fraudulence. Statistically, it is bound to produce superb success rates; for instance, in the case of oat-cell lung cancer, if all the patients said, "The doctor has given me three months," then even if the clinic does nothing to alter the course of the disease, approximately 75 per cent of the patients will survive longer than six months. Without doing anything at all, then, this clinic could report a success rate of 75 per cent.

Selective recall can affect the patient's interpretation not only of the prognosis, but also of the diagnosis itself.

> Harriet Thomas believes she owes her life to an iridologist. She had had cancer of the bowel and was told by her gastroenterologist that she needed surgery. The diagnosis was suggested by a barium X-ray and was confirmed by a sigmoidoscopy (in which a tube is inserted into the rectum, and a small biopsy is taken). She decided to ignore the specialist's recommendation for surgery and instead went to see an iridologist who confirmed the diagnosis of bowel cancer—without having heard that diagnosis or the symptoms from Harriet herself. The iridologist told her to make certain changes in her diet and to take certain remedies. Harriet has been following that advice now for seven years and is completely well. She never went back to see her gastroenterologist but feels that she is completely cured of her cancer and attributes the cure to the complementary practitioners.

At first sight, this story has all the elements of a miracle cure. After all, the patient had been seen by a conventional gastroenterologist and he had taken a piece of the tumour and had told her it was cancer. Everyone knows that cancer very rarely disappears of its own accord; therefore, it must be the case that the diet cured the cancer.

The actual situation was somewhat less dramatic. Harriet had not had a cancer of the bowel; she had a benign tumour called a polyp. There are many different kinds of polyp, and they are categorized on their form (some are frond-like, some are stumpy and some are tubular). Many studies following hundreds of patients for years suggest that all benign polyps can occasionally turn malignant (into cancer, in other words); the risk varies with the type of the polyp and the size. The tubular kind have the lowest risk; if the polyp is narrower than a centimetre, the risk of later developing bowel cancer is approximately 1 per cent. If the polyp is the stumpy kind and if it's larger than five centimetres, the subsequent risk is about 53 per cent.[7] As it happened, Harriet had the stumpy kind of polyp and the largest of her polyps measured under two centimetres. The risk of subsequent development of cancer in Harriet's situation is approximately 10 per cent. Her doctor thinks he told Harriet that she had a polyp that could be premalignant and if it was not removed there was a chance it would later develop into cancer. Harriet thought she was told she had cancer. Because the original interview seven years ago was not tape-recorded, we shall never know the exact truth of the interview—but the outcome is easy to see. The doctor thought he'd told the patient she had a risk of cancer; the patient thought the doctor had said she *had* cancer.

This story is not meant to insult or undermine either the doctor or Harriet. But it does show how easy it is to misunderstand the situation, particularly when a serious diagnosis such as potential cancer is involved, and how careful the professionals have to be to make sure the patients understand the situation correctly. However, the story also shows that a misunderstanding on a rather technical point of interpretation—albeit a very important one—can create the impression that diet can cure bowel cancer.

SIMULTANEOUS CONVENTIONAL TREATMENT

Of all the possible explanations of an apparent miraculous response to complementary medicine, perhaps the rarest—but still a very important reason—is that the patient was taking conventional therapy at the same time, but did not mention it, did not attach any importance to it or, sometimes, didn't realize what it was.

Penny Brohn is one of the four founders of the famous Bristol Cancer Help Centre; a major part of her motivation in starting the centre and providing complementary medicine techniques for cancer patients was her own experience with breast cancer.

She wrote a best-selling book, *Gentle Giants*,[8] which detailed her own struggles with the original breast cancer, its recurrence four years later and the various complementary approaches that she tried. In this detailed and fluent book, she describes in depth her moments of despair and doubt and her mixed feelings as she sought different opinions in different parts of the world. Two of the people that she describes as gentle giants are Dr. Josef Issels of Bavaria and Dr. Ernesto Contreras of Mexico, each well known in his own right as a complementary practitioner. In *Gentle Giants*, Penny Brohn sets out the details of a large range of complementary therapies. Over the course of many pages, she describes and discusses immunotherapy, detoxification, dry body rubs, venous oxygenation (in which blood is taken, oxygenated and returned to the patient's veins), pyrogen-induced fevers, several different diets, negative ionization, electric currents through the teeth, biofeedback, homeopathic remedies, coffee enemas, laetrile, iscadore, acupuncture and several different kinds of meditation and attitude modification. She records her dismay when the breast cancer recurred and the surprise and astonishment of her conventional doctors as the recurrent cancer began to shrink despite the fact that she had refused to have radiotherapy. Although there are no claims of miracles, there are many references to how surprising the remission was, and the reader is left with a very strong impression that the reversal of the progress of the breast cancer must in some way be related to the many complementary treatments that take up so much of the book. Even after careful scrutiny, the book appears to be detailing a triumph of unconventional medicine.

There are only six sentences in the whole book that give the real answer. When the cancer recurred, the recurrence was tested and was found to contain estrogen-receptors; the results of the test suggested a high likelihood of the cancer regressing when treated with hormone therapy. Her doctors recommended the hormonal anti-cancer drug tamoxifen and Brohn checked it out with Dr. Contreras. Brohn states that after much deliberation she decided to take the drug but she never mentions it again in the rest of the book.

When asked about this specific point in an interview, she replied that in fact she had taken the drug for many years, starting at the time of the recurrence of the cancer. Since tamoxifen is effective in approximately 60 per cent of hormone-sensitive breast cancers, nobody (including her doctors) should have been the least bit surprised that the recurrence shrank while she continued to take the most active conventional anti-cancer drug.

Brohn did not deny in her book that she took the drug, but even with the keenest eye, it is difficult for a reader to see that she continued on it while she also tried various diets and complementary medicines. Most readers of her book are left with the firm impression that her cancer was cured in a mysterious and baffling way, presumably attributable to the diets and other remedies. *Gentle Giants* is a widely read and influential book, and yet the central theme of it—that unconventional remedies may defeat cancer—is based on an under-emphasis of the crucial role of conventional treatment. In Brohn's list of nine Gentle Giants (comprising seven doctors, a vicar and her husband) at the front of the book, the drug tamoxifen, which is thoroughly gentle and acts like a giant in two-thirds of cases, doesn't even get a credit.

We were surprised when we unearthed the facts of this story. The Bristol Cancer Help Centre is known all over the world, partly because of its championing of holistic and complementary medicine for cancer patients (a function that it performs faultlessly and admirably) and partly because it received official recognition when it was opened by the Prince of Wales. Furthermore, Penny Brohn, as co-founder of the centre, has been strongly identified with all its objectives and aspirations and has constantly referred to her own battle as an example of what can be achieved. While her own odyssey is really quite remarkable and insightful in its own right (and as a description of the personal difficulties and exigencies of breast cancer, it should be recommended reading for everyone), quite clearly it is not a testament to the efficacy of complementary therapy in cancer but, if anything, underlines the importance of tamoxifen as well as caring.

In other cases, it is not the patient whose interpretation or emphasis of the situation is at fault, but the doctor's. The following story concerns a patient seen by one of us (R.B.).

Mrs. Turner had advanced cancer of the endometrium (womb). She had had radiotherapy some two years previously and had been well until the cancer had recurred in her pelvis, causing her some moderate pain and discomfort. She could not face the prospect of conventional chemotherapy, so she decided to go to a physician who specialized in complementary medicine. She was assured that she would not be given any conventional chemotherapy and was started on a variety of unconventional remedies, including some enzymes and doses of a drug that is supposed to work by altering the cancer cells' ability to handle sugar. Mrs. Turner came to our clinic for advice about pain control since the unconventional treatment did not seem to be working well after many weeks of injections. She and her husband brought with them a list of the medicines that she had been given. This list was given to the patient only because this particular physician worked outside the free provincial health service, and so the patient had to pay for her own drugs. Hence she was given an itemized bill.

When she gave me the lists, it was immediately apparent that among the unconventional medications, Mrs. Turner had been given standard chemotherapy on four out of ten occasions. In particular, she recalled that after the last injection, she felt particularly nauseous and could not understand why.

When I pointed out that she had been given chemotherapy (taking the discussion along very gently and cautiously), Mr. and Mrs. Turner were quite shocked. It had never been mentioned or even hinted that standard chemotherapy might be given and they both felt that they had been exploited and to some extent betrayed.

In Mrs. Turner's case, the shock, disappointment and anger were temporary, but she might have left with a very misleading impression of alternative medicine. Had her disease responded to the injections, she and her husband (as they said in an interview) would have both believed that alternative therapy was effective against endometrial cancer and would undoubtedly have recommended it to anyone they knew in the same position.

Conclusion: The Value of Optimism

To some extent it is possible, even likely, that these explanations of apparent miracles may cause distress and dismay, particularly to patients who have gained a great deal of comfort from the belief that miracle cures are possible. So we have to be clear about what we are implying here. We are not saying that there is no such thing as a miracle cure. What we are saying is that, in many cases, the apparent miracle has a more everyday explanation. In many examples, the data are simply unavailable and cannot be checked and verified (a situation we encountered many times in the research for this book). Often when they are available, the facts show that the disease would have recovered by itself, was subject to natural fluctuations or was misunderstood by the patient or by the doctor. In considering the likelihood of miracles, the philosopher David Hume (1711–76) wrote words that have been quoted and requoted over the last hundred years because they embody a piece of wisdom, a tool for analysis, that is still useful as we look at unusual claims about how the world works:

> The plain consequence is (and it is a general maxim worthy of our attention) "No testimony is sufficient to establish a miracle, unless the testimony be of such a kind, that its falsehood would be more miraculous than the fact which it endeavours to establish." ... When anyone tells me, that he saw a dead man restored to life, I immediately consider it with myself, whether it be more probable, that this person should either deceive or be deceived, or that the fact, which he relates, should really have happened. I weigh the one miracle against the other; and according to the superiority, which I discover, I pronounce my decision, and always reject the greater miracle.[9]

As Hume suggested, perhaps we should accept a phenomenon as a miracle only when the evidence for it is so strong that for the evidence to be wrong would be more miraculous than the fact it is trying to establish. If we are to accept fully that the animal in the garden is a unicorn, we need photographs from every angle to prove that it wasn't a goat seen from the side.

It is true that miracle stories such as the ones above do bring valuable messages of hope and potential triumph to some people, but they bring other messages to others. Claims of miracle cures may sometimes delude potential patients, raising false and fierce hopes, followed by bitter disappointment when those hopes are not realized. Miracle stories thus have side effects. They draw patients to try treatments that may consume much of their time, energy, money and hope and leave them poorer in all of them.

There is another point to be made about the popularity and currency of stories of surprising recoveries. It is often said that there are so many thousands of stories of miracle cures that the sheer weight of numbers must carry some credence. Surely, the argument goes, such a vast number of people cannot all be wrong or misled. However, the popularity of a belief is not, in itself, proof of its reality. For example, there are now millions of recorded sightings of unidentified flying objects, adduced as evidence of visits from alien beings. As with miracle cures, there are many possible explanations (weather balloons, reflections from airplane fuselages, objects falling from conventional planes, bright planets and so on). The number of documented sightings of UFOs does not prove that they really exist, but it does attest to the tremendous power and desire of our species to believe in them. In New York, there is a support group for people who are certain that they have been kidnapped by aliens and kept inside their spaceships for hours or even days. Some of the members of the group say that this happened to them more than a dozen times. The very existence of that support group shows that people are prepared to lend credence to the idea. The number of believers attests to the importance and the power of the belief among humans—it does not, in itself, prove that what we wish to believe in definitely exists.

In pursuing the truth, we may seem to be removing a source of comfort and solace. But finding out the facts should not and does not destroy the meaning of hope or the value of a positive outlook. In fact, as we shall see in the next chapter, a positive outlook and belief in the treatment may reduce the intensity of almost any bodily symptom even if it has no effect on an underlying disease.

8. Getting Better or Feeling Better

*The word "just" should never have been allowed
into the phrase "just the placebo effect."*

Feeling Better

So far we've seen some ways in which a patient's improvement might not be due to the treatment, but may be attributed to natural variations in the disease or to misinterpretation of the situation by the patient or by the doctor. Now we can move on to consider situations in which the patient feels better but the medical facts suggest that the underlying disease or condition is not improving. In some respects, the difference between feeling better and getting better is at the very centre of this whole investigation, and perhaps this is the most important (it's certainly the longest) chapter in the book, since it deals with the different ways in which healers, patients and observers regard the outcome of therapy. What might be seen as failure of treatment to an outsider might easily be regarded as a dramatic success to both the patient and the healer. Here's a clinical example:

Evelyn White was a patient with advanced recurrent breast cancer. The tumour had recurred in the left armpit and above the left clavicle and had blocked the lymphatic channels of her arm so that it had become swollen. There had been a temporary response to the first chemotherapy we had tried, but a few months later the disease became progressive again, and we suggested a second type of chemotherapy.

Mrs. White was unenthusiastic about the second-line chemotherapy and wanted to try a complementary medication called Cancell. I agreed to let her try and asked her to keep seeing me regularly so that I could assess her progress and perhaps offer symptomatic therapy if required. She visited every two weeks. Over a period of two months or so, she told me that her left arm was definitely less swollen and felt more comfortable and less tight. At each visit I measured the girth of the arm (at exactly the same place to avoid errors) and found that it was actually becoming more swollen. She asked me not to tell her what the measurements were and I honoured her request. She gradually became more ill as the disease progressed, but even at the end of her life she was convinced that the Cancell had done something for her. None of us argued with her—simply the subjective feeling that her arm was improving had given her a psychological boost that it would have been heartless (and pointless) to destroy.

Why did Mrs. White feel better? How could she feel that her arm was getting smaller and less tight, when it was actually getting bigger? In other words, how could she be feeling better while her tumour was getting worse? At a superficial level, one might be tempted to call this "self-delusion" or say that she was capable of "kidding herself." In some respects, this might be true, but there is much more to it than that. In fact, something happened during Mrs. White's interactions with her Cancell healer that changed her perception of her symptoms. She definitely was not *getting* better, but equally as definitely, she was *feeling* better. The power of the mind was able to change the severity of her symptoms as she experienced them. This is one way in which mental attitudes and attributes affect the way in which patients think about their physical or psychological problems and also change the way in which they tell other people about them. Because a patient's view of the situation and his or her hopes, fears or expectations can so drastically affect the outcome from their point of view, it's extremely important to know something about this interaction before trying to decide whether a treatment really works.

THE PLACEBO EFFECT

In medicine, there is a phrase for describing the way in which a person's expectations of a treatment alter the way the patient perceives the effect of the treatment. The phrase is "the placebo effect," and it really means the incidental—and sometimes accidental—useful effects of the whole intervention. The patient's expectations and reactions can be altered by anything associated with the treatment: the authority or humanity of the doctor, the calm of the consulting room, the receptionist, the fish tank in the waiting room, the colour of the tablets, the taste of the mixture, the ritual of taking the treatment or even the occult power of a totally illegible prescription written partly in Latin.

In other words, the placebo effect is "any useful effects accompanying some form of treatment that are not directly due to the treatment itself acting on the disease or the patient."[1] This clinical anecdote illustrates that sometimes even the doctor may not be fully aware of what is happening.

Peter Carol was a drummer with a British rock group that had become internationally famous. At the age of 21 he had a large personal fortune and was heavily addicted to heroin. He had made several attempts at withdrawing from heroin, but had suffered very badly from withdrawal symptoms each time and had gone back on the drug. I really don't know why he came to our little National Health hospital, or why, having come there he stayed; but he did.

I was a houseman (intern) at the time and I'd been medically qualified for all of two months. I felt totally ignorant and inept (justifiably, as it turned out). However, I really liked Peter and enjoyed talking to him and listening to him. One night I was called to the ward because he was going through an acute withdrawal attack. He was sweating and coughing but above all he said he felt that his mind was flying apart and that he was unbearably frenzied and twitchy. He thought he would have a complete breakdown if I didn't get him some tranquillizers immediately. I noted from his medical chart that he had been receiving massive doses of tranquillizers, including big doses of chlorpromazine and diazepam (Valium) by injection.

I sat and talked to him for about half an hour. He begged for large doses of tranquillizers but without my resident to supervise me, I felt far too scared to give him big doses of anything. In the end, with much trepidation, I prescribed a single tablet of two milligrams of Valium—

about the lowest dose there is. To my utter amazement (and probably to Peter's as well), he settled down in a few minutes and went to sleep peacefully.

The following morning, my resident laughed himself sick at what I had done. He pointed to the large doses of tranquillizers that had been needed before and told me (quite nicely but firmly) that I had no idea what I was doing. I agreed, and in fact, at the time, he was right—I had no idea what I was doing. It was only 20 years later that I realized that what I had done was a combination of psychotherapy and the placebo effect. And it worked beautifully.

Since the placebo effect is a crucial part of explaining why some patients feel better when they may not actually be getting better, it is worth spending some time examining it. Before we start that discussion, however, it is important to point out that other factors may make patients feel better without any placebo effect. For instance, psychotherapy, counselling, or psychiatric consultations may all have profound and long-lasting effects on a patient and her or his symptoms. But these are direct effects of the treatment that has been designed and administered specifically to improve the condition; they are not accidental or incidental side effects, and therefore they do not come within the definition of placebo effects.

The last two or three decades have seen a great deal of research into the placebo effect. And even though at first sight it seems to be mysterious, what we know of it makes it one of the most important—and perhaps most under-used—phenomena of medicine and healing.

The placebo effect had been studied occasionally for decades, but it really came into the foreground of medical research during the 1950s, and one of the significant studies that brought the placebo effect into the spotlight was an investigation of a new operation for angina.

Angina is pain arising from the heart when the cardiac muscle does not get enough oxygen for its needs. The commonest cause is a reduction in blood supply to the heart muscle due to narrowing of the coronary arteries by atherosclerosis. The standard first-line treatment for decades was (and still is) nitroglycerin tablets, which produce quick but brief relief of the pain. Early in the 1950s, some physicians in Italy had the idea that more blood might be diverted into the coronary arteries if some of the alternative pathways were closed down, reducing, as it were, the range of places to which the blood might flow.[2] The largest arteries in the area are the two internal mammary arteries that carry blood to the chest wall. An operation was devised in which an incision was made in the chest wall and the internal mammary arteries were tied off (ligated), resulting—it was hoped—in an increased flow of blood to the heart and a reduction in the angina pain.[3]

The operation was a success. After the operation, many patients experienced a considerable decrease in their angina pain, to the delight of both surgeons and patients. Despite everyone's satisfaction, it was generally acknowledged that no one knew precisely *how* the operation worked and nobody had conclusively demonstrated that the hoped-for diversion of blood to the heart did really happen. (It was known, for instance, that the operation didn't work when done on dogs.[4])

So in the late 1950s, two groups of researchers decided to look at the effects of this operation in greater detail and work out what was going on. The two groups carried out studies that would probably be forbidden by current ethical guidelines today but that were perfectly acceptable at the time. Patients with angina were randomly divided into two groups. One group got the standard internal mammary artery ligation operation. The other group, however, got a "sham" operation in which the chest wall incision was made but the internal mammary artery was left untouched. None of the patients knew the precise nature of the research study and none of the doctors who assessed the patients after surgery knew which operation had been performed.

The results of these studies were quite clear—and very upsetting for thoracic surgeons. The operation improved the pain, but it had nothing to do with the actual ligation of the internal mammary arteries. In one study, both groups reported the same subjective improvement after surgery (32 per cent average improvement in the group who had had the real surgery and 42 per cent improvement in the group that had had the sham operation).[5] Both groups also reported the same effect on their need for nitroglycerin tablets; the group who had the real operation decreased their daily consumption by 34 per cent while the "sham operation" patients reduced their dose by 42 per cent. But despite the fact that these patients felt better, there was very little improvement in objective measurements—the average improvement in the exercise they could perform was only one minute or so.

The second study produced similar results; the patients who had had the real operation all reported some improvement in the angina pain lasting in most cases for many months (90 to 100 per cent improvement in a third of the cases).[6] However, in the smaller group who had had the sham operation, all of them also reported a marked subjective improvement with decreased pain and decreased need for nitroglycerin.

The results of these studies caused a considerable stir. It was quite clear that the operation was beneficial for reducing angina, but equally clear that the act of tying off the internal mammary artery (the whole point of the operation in the first place) had nothing to do with the success of the procedure. Furthermore, it was obvious that patients could feel very much better (with less pain and decreased need for tablets) but could still have exactly the same objective problems (reduced ability to exercise and abnormal ECGs during exertion). The patients felt better but weren't getting better, and what made them feel better was "something that goes with having an operation on the chest," not the tying off of the internal mammary arteries. For want of a better phrase, "the placebo effect" gradually found its way into currency.

We now know that the placebo effect can cause an improvement in almost any bodily symptom, including pain, sleeplessness, nausea, and depression, and there is even a single reported case in which injections of placebo caused a documented regression of lymphoma. Overall, the placebo effect seems to produce an improvement in symptoms in at least one-third[7] of all patients and, in some series, up to 60 per cent.[8]

Placebo effects on symptoms

We now know that almost any physical or psychological symptom can be altered by placebo effects; in other words, every symptom can be modified in some patients by what the patient is expecting or how the patient perceives the treatment.

There are quite literally thousands of examples. Perhaps the easiest ones to understand are those to do with pain. A typical study might go like this. You take a group of patients with pain—say, patients recovering from a minor operation—and you tell them that you are trying out a new painkiller. You tell the patients that they will be given a tablet that might be the new painkiller or it might be a placebo (explaining that a placebo is a tablet that has nothing active in it at all). If they agree to enter the study after you've explained it properly (i.e., if they have given informed consent), then you organize it so that half the patients get the new painkiller, and the other half get the placebo. Let's say that 60 per cent of the patients who get the new painkiller report complete relief of pain after an hour. However, about 30 per cent of the patients who get the placebo will also report complete pain relief. Simply telling someone that they *might* get pain relief will reduce the pain they experience for a certain group of patients.

The same is true of many other symptoms—patients go to sleep when given a placebo that they think might be a sleeping tablet. Anxiety and depression can both respond to placebo treatment. It works for nausea, too; patients experience less nausea when they are given a tablet or injection that they have been told might be an antinauseant. The same effect has been recorded in a vast range of other symptoms—constipation, stiffness of joints, range of movement of limbs, itching, sexual function, breathlessness and so on.

What does this mean? Does it mean that humans are gullible and can be fooled into anything? Not really. What it means is that the conscious mind can override a vast range of bodily experiences. Perhaps this isn't as surprising as it seems; after all, our conscious minds cause all kind of physical effects—we can put our pulse rates up by watching horror movies, we can feel nauseated by experiencing a bad smell or seeing something upsetting and we can become sexually excited by erotic pictures or books (or even by phone calls, apparently). Therefore, we can see that how a patient reports a symptom is subject to considerable influence from the conscious mind—which is one of the ways in which somebody can feel better, without actually getting better.

A possible mechanism of action

Much research into the power of the placebo has been carried out in recent years but apart from demonstrating that it happens, and the conditions that favour its creation, there is no all-embracing theory of how a combination of externally caused mental phenomena lead to a reduction in pain, nausea, insomnia and so on. There are some clues—particularly as to one possible mechanism for the placebo action on pain. The hypothesis concerns substances produced inside the brain that reduce pain under certain circumstances. These chemicals are called endorphins and are produced by the brain under circumstances of extreme stress, which accounts for how soldiers can carry on fighting after a wound and feel no pain until after the battle. In 1978, one study showed that the placebo effect on pain could be switched off by a substance called naloxone, which antagonizes the pain-killing action of morphine and endorphins.[9] In other words, it's possible that the placebo effect on pain is partly accounted for by the brain producing endorphins in response to the expectations of the treatment. There is some controversy about this interpretation, and it's possible that this mechanism is only partial—if it's real—and would not account for the placebo effect on other symptoms.

But even if we can't—in the current state of knowledge—explain exactly how placebos work, that may not matter that much. There may be no need for a very complicated theory, on the basis that all the events that are wrapped up in the placebo effect are mental events—they use the same currency. Pain is a set of nerve messages to a receptive brain. Why shouldn't another set of nerve messages, embodying beliefs and expectations, interact in some way to diminish or change the coding of the messages so that they mean something different—less pain, for example?

Perhaps we shouldn't be too hypnotized by the apparently objective and factual nature of symptoms, compared to patients' verbal reports of what they're feeling. They are all the same thing; when someone says he or she has an itch or a pain or a feeling of nausea, he or she is still only expressing verbally an impression of a bodily symptom. The central nervous system receives impulses from the body, and the messages are interpreted by the conscious brain into language that seems appropriate. The philosopher J.J.C. Smart put this very neatly when he said, "When I 'report' a pain, I'm not really reporting anything—but am doing a sophisticated sort of wince."[10] Perhaps it shouldn't surprise us that all sorts of winces can be modified by the circumstances in which they occur.

Placebo effect as miracle cure

The placebo effect is one of the explanations of the miracle cures that are seen so commonly on stage or on television with evangelical or spiritual healers. Typically a patient comes on to the stage on crutches or in a wheelchair or with some other disability. The healer performs part of a ritual that incites the patient to more and more positive thinking about the disability. Then the patient—with all the audience also willing him or her out of the chair or whatever—makes an effort and stands up or walks a short distance to the untrammelled delight of all present.

A recent example was well documented when the American faith healer Maurice Cerullo visited Britain in 1992. At a healing ceremony at a big stadium in Earl's Court, one of the patients he called on to the stage was a young girl called Natalia Barned, who had a rare cancer with secondaries in the bones. The cancer had become resistant to chemotherapy and her conventional doctors were keeping her comfortable with powerful analgesics. On stage with Maurice Cerullo, she was encouraged to walk unassisted across the stage, which she did. Maurice told her that when she saw her conventional doctors next, they would tell her that the cancer in her bones had been cured. In fact, she did see the doctors shortly afterwards and no such cure had occurred. Natalia still required large doses of painkillers for the rest of her short life. The effect seen on stage was simply a temporary decrease in her perception of pain due to the effect of her conscious mind and will to improve.

This is not the only explanation of staged spiritual healing miracles—some are even simpler. At several faith healers' gatherings, it has been well documented that ordinary members of the audience are preselected by marshalls and taken to the front of the audience. They are offered a good view from seats that turn out to be wheelchairs (which the participants do not actually require). When the healer calls for everyone in a wheelchair to stand up and points at these members of the audience, they stand up (presumably because it is impossible and too embarrassing to explain to the cheering multitude that they didn't need the wheelchairs in the first place). Another miracle has been demonstrated.[11]

Placebo effect on lymphoma

So we can now see that placebo effects can influence almost any symptom—but can they also influence disease processes? In other words, can the mind alter the process of disease? As we shall discuss later, this is a very controversial issue in cancer, but as far as we are aware there is only one documented case in the world in which a proven tumour went into remission in response to a placebo.

In 1957 during a study of the psychological variables in patients with cancer, a bizarre case came to light.[12] A psychologist at the University of California in Los Angeles reported an extraordinary incident that today would be regarded as totally unethical and reprehensible, but that at the time was acceptable.

Mr. Wright was a patient with advanced lymphoma, which had become resistant to all palliative treatments available at the time. Because he was anaemic, his doctors did not attempt to use radiotherapy or the only chemotherapy agent available at that time, nitrogen mustard. The patient had "huge tumour masses, the size of oranges...in the neck, axillae, groin, chest and abdomen. The spleen and liver were enormous. The thoracic duct was obstructed and between one and two litres of milky fluid had to be drawn from his chest every other day."

He was bedridden and dependent on oxygen; the only treatment that helped was a sedative.

At that time, the American Medical Association was conducting a study into the usefulness of an alternative cancer remedy called krebiozen. In many ways, it had a similar reputation to laetrile in its heyday, and the medical association had allocated enough drug to treat 12 patients at the clinic where Mr. Wright was being treated. The study protocol specifically stipulated that patients would be considered for the study only if their life expectancy was at least three months. However, when Mr. Wright heard that krebiozen was available, he begged and pleaded to be put on the trial. Eventually, against his own better judgement, his doctor, Dr. Philip West, agreed and gave him the first dose of krebiozen on a Friday.

By the following Monday, Mr. Wright was a changed man. The tumour masses melted "like snowballs on a hot stove" and Mr. Wright "was walking around the ward, chatting happily with the nurses and spreading his message of good cheer to anyone who would listen."

Krebiozen seemed to work brilliantly, but only on one patient—Mr. Wright. In all other patients at that clinic, there were no other responses, and within two months, all the other clinics in the study reported no successes. Hearing all this bad news, Mr. Wright's faith waned, and after two months of near-perfect health, he relapsed to his original state.

At that point, Dr. West saw the opportunity to double-check the efficacy of krebiozen. He deliberately lied to the patient and told him that the newspapers were wrong and that the drugs seemed to be working after all. He then told him that the relapse was caused by the drug's short shelf life—it had deteriorated while standing in the pharmacy. Then Dr. West said that he had a new preparation of double-strength krebiozen that was due to arrive in two days. Two days later, with Mr. Wright in a state of eager anticipation, Dr. West started giving him injections of pure water.

The results of the water injections were even more dramatic than with the original krebiozen. His condition went into another remission, which lasted for another two months. At that time, the American Medical Association made a final announcement that nationwide tests had shown krebiozen to be useless. Mr. Wright was now readmitted to hospital, his faith gone and his last hope vanished. He succumbed in less than two days.

This case occurred 35 years ago in a climate in which doctors had greater freedom to do research that nowadays would be seen as unethical. It is an interesting example of useful data that could not have been obtained in any other way and clearly did not harm the patient. This seems to be the only recorded case in which a cancer patient was knowingly deceived and had a remission when given a placebo while the physician pretended it was something else. It's also very important to note that the diagnosis here was a lymphoma. Lymphomas are the kind of cancers that do fluctuate spontaneously, as we've already mentioned in the story of Audrey Parcell. There don't seem to be any other recorded cases in which a temporary remission was actually precipitated by a placebo. Perhaps the propensity of lymphomas to fluctuate may have been a major contributory factor, but this is certainly the most compelling (albeit the only) case of the placebo effect being associated with a remission in cancer.

Factors that affect the placebo response

It had always been assumed that the placebo effect was almost synonymous with "suggestion" and that it depended on the fact that the patient thought he or she was receiving (or at least might be receiving) active therapy. One study showed that the placebo effect worked even if the patients knew they were receiving an inert substance.[13] Fifteen patients in a psychiatric ward suffering from neurotic symptoms were asked to try a placebo by a doctor using a carefully composed script ("We feel that a so-called sugar pill may help you. Do you know what a sugar pill is? A sugar pill is a pill with no medicine in it at all. I think this pill will help you as it has helped so many others. Are you willing to try this pill?") Fourteen out of 15 patients agreed to take the sugar pill, and of those 14, 13 improved during the week of taking the sugar pills, some of them by a great deal and at least one, who had been suicidal, showed one of the most dramatic improvements of the whole group.

So the placebo effect is more than a deception or sleight of hand (or rather speech). It is a phenomenon that is clearly rooted in the human ability to believe in treatment and to perceive symptoms accordingly.

The placebo effect is also enhanced if the material that is used as an inactive substance has a side effect similar to the active (i.e., the sham treatment has none of the benefits but some of the side effects of the real treatment); for instance, drug investigators have used atropine as a placebo in a trial of antidepressants because it produces the side effect of dry mouth—as antidepressants do—but has no activity against the depression itself.[14]

The effect of the healer

There are many different factors that enhance the effect and strengthen the patient's belief that the treatment will work. One of these, paradoxically, is the strength of the doctor's belief. Several surveys of doctors' attitudes have shown that if the doctor is enthusiastic about a form of treatment, he or she will get better results than a sceptic will. The best illustration of this came from a review of the literature in angina; investigators re-examined studies that had used drugs later found to be ineffective. This meant that the early results must have been due to placebo effects. It was interesting to see that the initial reports—in the enthusiastic phase of the drug-doctor relationship—yielded 70 to 90 per cent effectiveness, whereas as enthusiasm waned, the effectiveness fell to the usual range for placebo responses—30 to 40 per cent.[15]

William Silverman, a distinguished paediatrician who has spent a lifetime analyzing the pitfalls of over-confidence among doctors convinced that their pet treatments worked, cites the following astonishing instance. A remarkable example of the complex interactions in medical treatment was cited by Stewart Wolf of the University of Oklahoma. He told of a patient with long-standing and almost continuous asthma who obtained no relief from a series of drugs tried by the treating doctor. When an experimental drug with a high promise of effectiveness became available, a supply was obtained by the doctor. The new drug relieved the asthmatic symptoms immediately. When it was stopped, the asthma returned. The doctor substituted a placebo without the patient's knowledge; this failed to relieve symptoms. Shifts from new drug to placebo and back again were tried several times with consistent results in favour of the experimental agent. When the pharmaceutical company was approached for an additional supply, the doctor was amazed to learn that, because of worry about unjustified claims, the company had, in this instance, provided only a placebo preparation. The patient had never received an active drug at all.

Clearly, in this case, the only factor that could have caused the patient's alternation between symptoms and no symptoms—since one placebo alternated with another—was the influence of the doctor's belief that one of the placebos was actually an active preparation.

The placebo effect in active treatments

So far we've been discussing the placebo effect as it is seen with sham (or "dummy") treatments. But there is a placebo effect even in treatments that are known to be active. This point was neatly made by Socrates:

> I said that the cure itself is a certain leaf, but in addition to the drug, there is a certain charm, which if someone chants when he makes use of it, the medicine altogether restores him to health, but without the charm there is no profit from the leaf.[16]

The main surgical treatment of angina nowadays is an operation called coronary-artery bypass-graft (CABG) in which lengths of "spare" vein are taken from the leg and stitched to the coronary arteries to act as bypass channels to get past the blocked area. This operation has been shown to improve survival when the blockage is either very widespread or in a dangerous position—if all three coronary arteries are blocked or if a crucial supply vessel called the left main stem is blocked. In those circumstances, the operation prolongs the survival of patients who have surgery (compared to those who don't). But these patients represent only a small proportion of the total number of patients with angina. For the remainder of the patients, the operation produces an impressive decrease in the angina pain but doesn't improve survival.

So far so good—the operation reduces symptoms in most patients and improves survival in a few. But then a most curious anomaly was found. The effect of the graft can be assessed by repeating angiography (injection of dye into the blood vessels) to check that the grafts are open and allowing blood flow. In a number of patients, it was found that some time after surgery the grafts themselves had blocked up and there was no blood flow through them.[17] Quite surprisingly, many of these patients still experienced relief of the angina pain. The treatment that usually worked had a placebo effect on the patients for whom it didn't work.

THE GOLD STANDARD

The fact that some patients—perhaps a third of them or more—will notice some improvement in their condition despite the fact that they have not received any active treatment makes it difficult to know what to believe. If we also take into account all the various confounding factors mentioned in the last chapter—fluctuations in the disease, self-limiting conditions, spontaneous remissions and so on—it might seem almost impossible to decide whether a treatment is really working, and whom to believe.

Fortunately, there are techniques that are now widely accepted and practised that can tell us whether the claims for a form of treatment are valid or not, and whether we can really believe any particular set of results. That process—of trying to assay the amount of truth in a set of observations—is a bit like taking a lump of gold ore to an assay office. You go in with a lump of material and the man compares the weight and size of your lump with "the gold standard"—the figure you'd get if the lump was pure gold. There is a very similar process in analysis results of experiments, and at the end of the procedure, it's possible to have a fairly accurate idea of how much of the data is true and believable. This assaying process has been applied over the centuries to many different fields, some of which have emerged with good marks and have earned the title of science (astronomy, physics, chemistry, biology and so on) while others have been shown to be anecdotes strung together with wishful thinking or sometimes deception (alchemy, astrology, phrenology and so on). When this assaying process has been applied to clinical medicine, it can be used to decide whether the results of a treatment are really believable.

It has to be said, though, that for centuries, many people (doctors included) thought you didn't need any fancy techniques or analyses to tell you whether a particular medical procedure was right or wrong. Most people thought you could tell simply by looking at it. Sadly, however, it turns out that most people (including most doctors) are not actually very good at "simply looking at" research and judging its value by appearances only.

It can't be right, it looks wrong

The history of conventional medicine is littered with the wrecks of great therapies that looked promising and never made the grade. Just as frequently, therapies that we now regard as standard and routine were ridiculed when they were first introduced.

In the first category, we can include radical mastectomy for breast cancer (the extensive operation achieved no better results than the far less mutilating simple mastectomy or even lumpectomy), immune-therapy (with BCG vaccination) for the treatment of leukaemia, transfusions of white cells for patients whose own white cells are very low and who have got a fever (it doesn't help), routine and regular testing for blood in the stool (to detect early bowel cancer), carotid endarterectomy (coring out the centre of furred-up carotid arteries) for strokes (which it does not prevent), chest X-rays on the whole population to detect very early cancer or TB and so on.

All these ideas seemed right and appropriate at the time. They went through a phase of wide acceptance, followed by a phase of testing during which the results that emerged simply weren't good enough. So these are breakthroughs that never broke through.

On the other hand, there is an equally large number of therapies we now accept as routine that almost caused riots when they were first introduced. Sigmund Freud was ostracized when he dared to suggest that some patients' physical symptoms arose from past psychological problems. Dr. Ignatz Semmelweiss was persecuted and actually died in a psychiatric asylum as a result of the opprobrium he drew for suggesting that puerperal (childbed) fever in women was caused by something on the hands of the medical students who had come to the ward straight from the post-mortem room. Werner Forssmann, the first brave physician who pushed a rubber tube into the veins of his own arm and back into his heart, was almost expelled from his hospital. The use of massive doses of anti-cancer drugs and rescuing the patient by saving some of his or her bone marrow before the therapy and giving it back afterwards was ignored totally when it was first reported in 1961.[18]

Looking superficially at these examples, we can safely conclude that we can make no safe conclusions about the value of a treatment simply by looking at it superficially. Appearances can clearly be deceptive. However, we should add that if appearances cannot be relied on to rule out a form of therapy, nor can they be relied on to validate it. A number of believers in iridology, for example, point out that representing the entire body in the iris is not really different from acupuncture in which the entire body is represented on the skin.

The argument is akin to "They all laughed at Christopher Columbus...." In other words, since the powers that be ridiculed someone who discovered America (albeit accidentally), anyone who is similarly ridiculed must have made a similarly important discovery. However, it needs to be stressed that if appearances are unreliable, they are unreliable—no useful information can be obtained from them. They may indeed have laughed at Christopher Columbus but some of them also laughed at Hieronymous Thompson who said he could turn grass into milk without a cow.[19] A radionics box may look just like a skin-resistance meter (which measures sweat as a parameter of sympathetic nerve activity), but that doesn't necessarily prove that the radionics box's measurements are reliable or valid. And at the other end of the scale, unimpressive appearances don't tell us anything either. A consultant neurologist may use a cheap red-headed pin to test for visual problems in a patient on chloroquine. The fact that the pin costs five cents doesn't undermine the value or the reliability of the test (or of the consultant).

So, appearances are only appearances, and if they are deceptive, then what criterion would do instead? Many people set a great deal of store on whether the technique or results have been published in an established journal. For the last century or so, there have been many eminent respectable medical journals with representatives of eminently respectable medical establishments on their eminent and respectable editorial boards. By and large, these journals use the system of peer review to decide whether an article is worthy of publication. Peer review means that the submitted article is sent to three or four acknowledged international experts in the field, who assess the paper and inform the editor whether they think the paper cuts the mustard. Generally this system works well. In the vast majority of cases, if an article has made it into the *New England Journal of Medicine*, or *The Lancet* or *Nature* or *Science*, you can believe it. Of course, there are the occasional exceptions. *The Lancet* once published an article from Spain about a new treatment for cancer called thioproline (Norgamem). The result is that the paper's claims proved to be unrepeatable, and the authors were never able to establish any efficacy of thioproline. More recently, Professor Jacques Benveniste and colleagues thought they had proved the basis of homeopathy by showing that very high dilutions of an antibody (containing no residual molecules of the original material) had an effect on white cells; their results were published in the prestigious, peer-reviewed journal, *Nature*. At a later investigation, it was reported that the Benveniste research team had not been including all results of consecutive experiments, but had thrown out some of the experiments when the results didn't fit.

Furthermore, publication in an established journal tends to be in line with the status quo. It's a self-preserving territory. As many pioneers have found (for example, in acupuncture), quite valid research may be rejected by eminent journals because there aren't any other articles on the same subject that it can be compared to. As with everything—from fashion to philosophy—it's very hard to be the first in a new field.

So if you can't always trust what the treatment looks like or the publication (or non-publication) in established journals, how *can* you know what to believe?

The coming of age of a science

We all think we know what a science is. Science is what is written in the newspapers under the heading "by our science correspondent." It's what scientists do, and scientists are people with wild staring eyes and no fashion sense who talk on news programs for seven seconds about the origins of the sun or the dangers of strawberry jam or the end of the human species or all three. In short, science is thoroughly believable and totally unintelligible.

Perhaps the most important part of that popular view of science is the part that says science is believable. Scientists say that the universe began with a big bang, and shock waves are still being detected in space that confirm that theory. Scientists say that Mars is uninhabitable. Scientists say that cigarette smoking causes most lung cancer. Scientists say that there is a hole in the ozone layer and that mankind's production of CFCs created it.

Why do we believe them? Why do we look at satellite photographs and believe that they show a thinned ozone layer? Or at cancer statistics and believe them? And if we believe all that without actually checking up on the ozone layer or outer space for ourselves, why shouldn't we also believe the man at the Annual Fair of Mystics who says that hanging a magic crystal in our window will keep us free of all known diseases?

Of course all belief is a matter of choice, so any person has the freedom to believe anything he or she likes. But observations that are part of something called a science share certain properties that make it easier for large numbers of people to accept them without having to check for themselves. A science means a body of knowledge that is objective—observations made by one person or group that can be repeated and verified by other people and other groups. If I measure the force of gravity at sea level in London, you'll get the same value as if you measure it at sea level in Venice or Martha's Vineyard. The speed of light will be the same (roughly) wherever it is measured and by whom. An ultrasound of a gallbladder with gallstones in it will look the same whether it is examined by a radiologist in Bradford, Bombay or Beijing. Science means the body of knowledge that we know (from the Latin word *scire* to know)—if it's science, it's fact (or is on the way to becoming fact).

Refutability: the benchmark of believable truth

So how do observations grow up into sciences? How do experiments go through the equivalent of the assay process and come out with a piece of paper stating how much gold is mixed in with the dross? The answer is based on a pattern to which everything that deserves the title science matches up, and anything that doesn't, doesn't. In a single sentence it can be boiled down to this: Before you can state something's correct, you have to try very hard to prove that it's wrong. The essence of a scientific process is the attempt at *disproving* the hypothesis. If you can't prove it's wrong when you have tried very hard, then perhaps—just perhaps—it's right.

At the moment, the word "science" has acquired a reputation it doesn't deserve. Many people believe that science is simply one of many possible ways of looking at things and that there are alternative ways we can choose if we wish to look at things differently. This often comes up in discussion of the findings of science, and it is bedevilled by the difference between what *science* says and what *scientists* say. To take a simple example: A scientist may say, "Lead in gas does not cause brain damage in children." "Science" will say a similar thing in a much more complicated way, beginning something like: "In a range of surveys of children who have been brought up in an area with lead levels derived from exhaust emissions...compared with children brought up in areas with lower lead levels...no significant difference was found between the two groups, p = .005."

Clearly there are similarities between the two statements, but there are also major differences. The first statement is easier for non-scientists to understand than the second. It is also more definite. As phrased, it is unambiguous; it cannot allow the possibility of lead in gas causing any brain damage at all in children. It is also general and all-encompassing; "children" means "all children everywhere," whereas the second statement is about a specific group of children, the ones in the study, and it tries to be as accurate as possible in what it says about them.

The problem is, because the first statement is memorable, shorter and easier to understand, it is the one that gets remembered and passed on more often than the second. But it is usually wrong. Truly scientific statements apply only to specific circumstances and events at specific times. To say "The sun rises every morning" is actually all right because it is true of every morning so far. To say "The sun always rises" is unsupportable by evidence. To say "On every morning so far observed by me (personal communication) the sun has risen" is about as near as we can get to a truthful statement by one individual. So "Homeopathy is good for migraine" is not nearly as scientific as "administering a homeopathic pill was followed by pain relief in ten cases of migraine." But even that is not ideal, unless we know how many cases it didn't relieve. If it relieved ten out of eleven, that's good news. If it relieved ten out of a thousand, it doesn't really give us much useful information about homeopathy.

Issues of what is scientific and what isn't have been a topic of much analysis in the first half of this century as philosophers have tried to wrestle with the dilemmas that occur when major beliefs about science turn out to be wrong or only partial. One of the most distinguished writers on this topic is Karl Popper, who provided a definition that is useful in analyzing new hypotheses about the world and deciding whether to take them seriously.

To simplify Popper, he says that in considering any hypothesis we should ask whether it is possible to think of some event that would refute it. "The sun always rises," for example, can be refuted by an event that is easy to imagine—waking up at 11 o'clock in the morning, looking out of the window and seeing the stars and the night sky (unless you are an inhabitant of Tromso.) "Aspirin is good for headaches" could be refuted if aspirin were given to a hundred people with headaches and did no good at all. It is possible to imagine a situation that would refute the hypothesis "A mass exerts a force on another mass." This would be refuted if you were to place two masses in a frictionless environment where there were no other forces acting on them, and they failed to move towards each other.

But now look at Galen's hypothesis, quoted earlier: "All who drink of this remedy recover in a short time, except those whom it does not help, who all die. Therefore, it is obvious that it fails only in incurable cases." To test this statement in the same way as the others, we should try to imagine a case that would refute it. This is not easy. If somebody drinks the remedy and recovers, that would confirm the statement, not refute it. If somebody drinks but dies, that is allowed for, since the person was obviously incurable, by the definition in the statement.

The significance of all this is that a statement is to be considered scientific only if we can think of a way of testing it by an experiment, i.e., creating the circumstances in which one possible outcome is the sort of refutation we've looked at above. If, whatever we do to test a statement, all possible outcomes of that process can only confirm it then it is not scientific.

This way of looking at the scientific method is called the hypothetico-deductive model because in order to support a hypothesis, you have to derive a deduction from it that is indisputably derived from the hypothesis and that can be tested. Then the deduction is tested. This means that no current scientific hypotheses (e.g., gravity, $e=mc^2$, evolution, DNA replication and so on) are actually proven. They are all awaiting possible refutation, but until someone comes along with a watertight experiment that disproves any of these hypotheses, we can accept them as working truths.

This, then, is the nature of real proof—there must be a refutable deduction derived from the hypothesis and it must be tested. We need to stress this point, because quite a lot of claims are made and supported without using this process, but using induction instead. To put it simply, "induction" means "you have an idea and grab any evidence that you can find to support it." Of course, most great ideas begin that way—presumably James Watt sat by his mother's kettle and reached his idea of steam power by a process of creative induction. But induction—however necessary in dreaming up an idea—is not enough to prove it.

A neat example of this was recently put forward by Professor Michael Baum.[20] Suppose a young mathematician suddenly thinks of a hypothesis that all odd numbers are prime numbers and cannot be divided by any other numbers. When the mathematician starts looking, he finds supporting evidence—1, 3 and 5 are all prime numbers. He looks for further evidence—7 is also a prime number. The theory is looking good. He has a problem with 9, but if he can dismiss that as experimental error, he's doing well through 11 and 13. This is (basically) inductive logic. If he wants to look at it scientifically, however, he would have to propose that there are no odd numbers that are not prime numbers—and he'd have to accept that 9, 15, 21, 25 and so on are not prime numbers and so refute his hypothesis.

This may seem like nit-picking and logic-chopping, but it really isn't. It tells us a way of deciding what we can really believe and what we can't. If there is a refutable deduction derived from the idea and if that deduction is tested and is not refuted, you can believe it (for the time being). If there is no refutable deduction, there is no proof. However high-falutin that may sound, it's tremendously important in looking at the results of medical treatment—in fact, if you ignore that rule, you can devise a treatment that works in every single case.

The infallible Freireich Experimental Plan

As an example of how, if we don't adopt the refutability principle, we can get in a tricky but familiar situation, here is the Freireich Experimental Plan, devised by a distinguished American cancer researcher, Emil J. Freireich III and published in the journal *Cancer Chemotherapy*. Freireich was clearly driven to write this by the succession of cancer therapies that were becoming publicized at the time, persuading some of his patients to question the harsh but effective conventional anti-cancer drugs that they were being prescribed. It is a masterful analysis of all medical treatment and how it can appear to be effective when it isn't necessarily so.

There are two essential requirements in the Freireich Experimental Plan (hereafter FEP). The first is a treatment of some sort. It doesn't have to be a drug—it could be a device, some kind of hand-waving, an age-old herb, an acupuncture needle. The second requirement is that whatever treatment is offered should be absolutely harmless. Starting from these two conditions, Freireich shows how any alternative therapy can be administered in such a way that any outcome can be interpreted as confirming its success, and no conceivable outcome could falsify it—heads I win, tails you lose.

The key factor in his analysis is the natural variability of almost all human diseases. The graph shows the typical course of a serious illness. Freireich points out that every disease, acute or chronic, has important periods of remission, the ups on the graph.

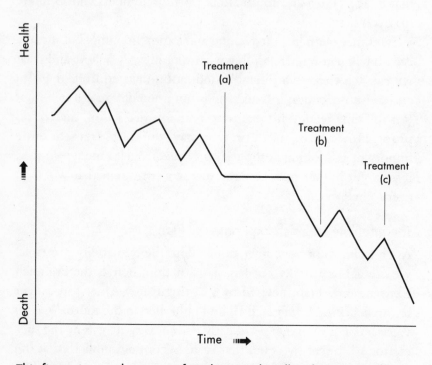

This figure is an adaptation of Emil Freireich's all-embracing explanation of how therapy can be demonstrated to work, whatever happens to the patient. The lines show the (hypothetical) progress of a disease that will ultimately bring about the patient's death. If the disease fluctuates, the healer can claim that any improvement is due to the therapy (providing the therapy itself is harmless). At any point, the patient's condition can only (a) stay the same, (b) improve or (c) get worse. For each of these outcomes, the treatment can be shown to be effective if the healer says (a) "The disease would be getting worse were it not for the treatment," (b) "the treatment is working" and (c) "You should have come to me sooner."

At those times the patient feels better than he has done for some time, and in fact he is physically better by all objective measurements. This is true even if there is an inexorable trend downward, and even truer, of course, in the case of diseases that are not potentially fatal. "There is no disease I know," says Freireich, "where inevitable and continuous progression is the universal characteristic." On the basis of these observations, Freireich has devised a set of rules for the would-be alternative therapist. The first rule is that treatment should be applied to a patient only after a period when he has been getting progressively worse (point A on the graph). If you give the treatment during an up (at point B) and the patient continues to improve, he can always say he would have got better anyway. But if treatment is applied when the patient is getting worse, four possible things could happen. First, the patient could start to improve. Natural variability will ensure that this possibility is always present. If it happens, it immediately "proves" that the treatment is effective. Second, the disease could stabilize. This also "proves" that the treatment is working, because it has arrested the disease. What is needed now, says Freireich, is a treatment of a higher dose, or for a longer period. This will, of course, cause no harm because the treatment is harmless. A third possibility is that the patient continues to get worse. However, the healer need not be at all put out by this, even if the patient is, because this can be taken to mean that the initial dosage was inadequate and must be stepped up, or that the treatment hasn't been administered for long enough. The fourth, and saddest, outcome is that the patient dies. The death has to be taken as an indication that the patient delayed consulting the healer for too long and the treatment was applied too late—"If only he'd come to me sooner."

So far so good. If you are a therapist following the Freireich Experimental Plan and have applied it to a number of patients, you will already have had some successes—the ones who started to get better. But you still have a number of patients who stayed the same or continued to get worse, whom you are continuing to treat.

It is now time to move on to a second phase. Here, the rule is to treat the patients who remain in the same way as you treated the patients in phase 1—applying your therapy only when they have got worse. There will be some more successes—because of the natural variability of disease—and there will be some patients who need to continue with more intensive treatment.

As you apply these procedures stage by stage, you will end up with two groups of patients—the ones who have shown objective improvement (thanks apparently to your treatment) and those who are dead, who can be excluded from your study because, in spite of all your efforts, their delay in seeking treatment meant that they were beyond saving.

There's a third and even more ingenious stage that helps to confirm the effectiveness of the treatment among those patients who are showing improvement. Once the patient improves, you must reduce the dose. This is then followed by two possible outcomes: (1) the patient continues to show improvement, which proves how effective the treatment has been, or (2) the patient's disease stabilizes or gets worse, which is also proof of the effectiveness of the treatment. In fact, it is a well-known principle of homeopathy that when you apply a remedy the patient will often get worse before improving, which is taken as an indication that the remedy is exactly right for the condition you are treating.

This last point is a reminder of where we started, with the question of the "scientific" nature of statements about treatments. Freireich's tongue-in-cheek analysis shows how it is possible to use a therapy in such a way that whatever the outcome, it can be taken as confirming the success of the therapy, or at least not refuting it. You cannot imagine any event during that patient's encounter with that therapy which would refute or disprove the effectiveness of the therapy. Similarly, with the last statement, about homeopathy, it plugs a hole through which the plausibility of the therapy would otherwise leak. If even "getting worse" is taken as a sign of success, the statement that homeopathy works can never be refuted.

Of course, some people may argue: "So what? It may be important to you that statements about a therapy are scientific but to me that doesn't matter. I don't care whether you can prove anything or not—I just believe that these things work, even if your science can't show it. There are more ways of looking at the world than through the myopic spectacles of science." People expressing such views don't realize that the scientific method is something that we ignore at our peril. It is the scientific method that leads us to decide whether to take an umbrella on a rainy day, walk across eight lanes of a busy motorway in rush hour or practise unsafe sex. These are all situations where inferences from existing evidence lead to beliefs about how the world works. To say that there are other paths to knowledge than science is like saying to your bank manager that you may appear to have an overdraft by his stuffy, narrow methods of calculating but with your rainbow-coloured, yin/yang "natural" sort of arithmetic, you believe that you are vastly in credit. You may be allowed to believe it, but you will be asked to take your account to a less scientific bank, if you can find one.

CLINICAL TRIALS

If we accept that it's the process of attempted refutability that turns a group of observations into a science, we now ought to find out whether medicine has been subjected to that analysis—and if so, what happened. Has clinical medicine made the grade and graduated as a science, or has it failed and been condemned to remain a collection of anecdotes and empirical observations?

First, we need to understand that the process of attempted refutation is much easier when the disease is a serious one.

If, for example, a disease is universally fatal—that is, if 100 per cent of all patients die of it—and if a treatment saves even a small number of lives (even as small a number as one, assuming the diagnosis is correct), the results are scientifically valid. That's why there are no early clinical trials of antibiotics in overwhelming infections. When streptomycin was first used in tuberculous meningitis, for instance, no clinical trial was needed. Tuberculous meningitis (infection with tuberculosis of the membranes around the brain, a rare but disastrous condition) had a mortality rate of 100 per cent. When streptomycin was first introduced and given by lumbar puncture to patients with this meningitis, patients began to survive the illness.

And small numbers proved the case—even two or three cases of proven tuberculous meningitis surviving after streptomycin were quite acceptable as scientific proof of the effectiveness of the therapy.

If proof is simple when the disease is serious, things become much more complex when the disease is less serious and the effects of treatment are less dramatic and occur only some of the time. This is when proper scientific tests are needed to find out if the treatment being given produces any genuine benefit, or if there are simply variations in the disease due to random chance.

The single most reliable way of testing a new therapy—and either proving its benefit or refuting it—is called the randomized clinical trial (or RCT), and it is the single most important method of putting medical practice through the hypothetico-deductive method of testing.

The idea of the randomized clinical trial is simple. Suppose you have what you think is a miraculous new treatment for a disease. You take a group of patients with that disease and give half of them the new treatment; you give the other half the standard routine treatment for that disease—assuming that they all agree to enter the trial in the first place.

The idea is to compare your new treatment with whatever the standard treatment is for that disease at the time. The group that receives your new treatment is usually called the treatment group or treatment arm of the trial, and the group that receives the standard therapy or the placebo is called the control group or control arm. If the condition is a headache and the usual treatment for a headache is aspirin, you give half the patients your new treatment and the control group gets aspirin. If the condition is something for which there is no effective standard treatment, you give the control group nothing—or rather, because of the placebo effect, you give them an inactive placebo that looks like your new treatment.

But, because you might be biased, and you might be tempted to put, let's say, patients who you think might do well into the new treatment group, and patients who you think might do badly into the other or control group, you assign the patients at random. It can be done with a computer program or a book of random numbers or a set of pre-assigned cards shuffled into random order or any of several other methods. Each patient receives what looks like the same treatment, which is identified only by a code number. The patients are assessed carefully and the symptoms or parameters of the disease are assessed as well as any possible side effects of the treatment. In a perfect trial, nobody will know who has received what until the trial is over and the code is broken. The object of the exercise is that nobody— not the patient, the doctor or anybody looking after the patient— should be able to influence the assignation of the patient into one group or the other, nor the way in which patients assess their treatment or symptoms (thus eliminating placebo effects).

If the trial is conducted correctly, at the end of it, the investigators will have a comparison between the new treatment and the control arm (the placebo group or the standard treatment group) and they will be able to say categorically that the new treatment (compared to the placebo or standard treatment) is better, worse or the same.

One of the most famous demonstrations of the value and use of a randomized clinical trial is in a condition that affects the eyes of newborn babies. In the 1940s, small or premature babies were being saved when in earlier eras they would have died. Doctors began to notice changes in their eyes. Some babies developed a disease behind the lens of the eye; uncontrolled growth of blood vessels gradually and tragically made the children become blind. The disease was named retrolental fibroplasia (RLF).[21] As medical understanding of the progress of the disease increased, it became possible to identify the earliest changes of RLF—in other words, to identify the RLF process as it began with the branching and sprouting of the blood vessels at the back of the eye. Because it was already known that steroids reduced the uncontrolled cell growth seen in blood vessels at the start of processes very similar to RLF, steroids (actually a steroid-releasing drug called ACTH) were tried. In one hospital in New York, 31 babies with early changes in RLF were given ACTH. Twenty-five of those babies recovered completely and were left with normal eyes. By contrast, at a nearby hospital, a group of seven babies with the early changes of RLF was observed and six of those seven eventually became blind.

These initial observations were very important. It seemed by comparing the two groups (at different hospitals) that ACTH reversed the early changes of RLF and saved the babies' vision. However, these were initial observations only, and everybody concerned wanted to *prove* that ACTH was effective treatment for RLF. A randomized trial was set up in which babies *at the same hospital* were to receive either ACTH or nothing. When the trial results were analyzed, it was found that ACTH made no difference to the RLF at all. Depending on how early the "early" changes were, a lot of the babies got better anyway, and of the others, the ACTH didn't slow down the progress of the RLF. In other words, the initial differences seen between the two groups of babies at the separate hospitals must have been due to something else—perhaps the "earliness" of the early changes.

This is a classic demonstration of why randomized clinical trials are so important. If the doctors had been using inductive reasoning only and had been satisfied with the initial observations at the two hospitals, they would have gone on to recommend to the whole world that the early changes of RLF should be treated with ACTH. That would have been a disaster. ACTH produces serious side effects in babies—problems in growth, in bone development and other side effects. Perhaps those serious side effects would have been acceptable compared to blindness (or perhaps not) but since the drugs didn't prevent blindness anyway, those side effects were completely unnecessary. The randomized clinical trial saved thousands of babies from dangerous ineffective treatment.

Since then, thousands of different types of procedures—drugs, operations, diagnostic tests and other techniques—have been tested with randomized clinical trials. At its best, and provided that it is repeated and confirmed, a randomized clinical trial can be used to change medical practice all over the world. One recent example is the treatment of early breast cancer. In just under half the cases of breast cancer in women, the lymph nodes in the armpit contain some cancer cells. In those cases, we know that the chance of recurrence is much higher than if the lymph nodes are uninvolved. In the mid-1960s, several doctors wondered whether the chance of recurrence could be decreased if the women were given treatment just after the operation—in other words, whether recurrence could be prevented before it actually happened.

With an idea like this, only a randomized clinical trial could give the answer. No amount of anecdotal evidence would do. The initial randomized clinical trial showed that treatment did work—it prevented recurrence in some of the patients (compared to no treatment in the control arm). The studies were repeated in a number of centres, and to confirm the various studies, a big analysis (called a meta-analysis) involving thousands of patients in those trials was performed. The results were entirely consistent; on average, about one-third of recurrences could be prevented by treatment, and giving treatment to node-positive patients is now the standard therapy all over the world.

The results of these—and all other—investigations are usually expressed in statistical terms, which tell us how certain we can be that the results are genuine. Unfortunately, the word "statistics" causes abreactions in most normal people—including eye-rolling, nausea, loss of consciousness and occasionally convulsions and coma. We shall therefore give a brief and entirely painless crash course in medical statistics—designed entirely for people who hate the idea of statistics (which includes most doctors).

A crash course in statistics

The whole purpose of statistics in medicine is to help us decide whether an effect that we are studying is a real effect or has happened by chance. It's as simple (and, in practice, as complex) as that.

Let's pick a theoretical example: Suppose you are trying to invent a cure for *digititis minimis*, a mythical and trivial inflammation of the little finger. Suppose that this disease gets better by itself in one-third of cases. Then suppose that you treat three cases of *digititis minimis* with your home remedy (betel juice and oil of squills), and all three patients get better. You rush to telephone the local newspaper, and you tell them (somewhat breathlessly) that your remedy has increased the cure rate from 33 per cent to 100 per cent. On a national scale, thousands of sufferers from epidemic *digititis minimis* can be saved from days of discomfort and can be back at the typewriter or piano immediately, vastly increasing the nation's output of typescript, "Chopsticks" and "Für Elise." You settle back in your chair and anticipate great wealth and renown—until you are telephoned by a statistician.

The statistician's job, as we've just said, is to find out how often a particular event could occur by chance. If *digititis* gets better anyway in one-third of cases, then, the statistician asks himself, how often will we see all three patients getting better in a random sample of three patients? To answer that question, he applies a set of mathematical tests to the figures and comes up with the answer. The answer in this case is 27 per cent of the time. "To put it simply," the statistician tells you, "if you took a hundred groups of three patients with *digititis* and gave them no treatment at all, with a spontaneous recovery rate of 33 per cent, most groups of three would happen to have one or two recoverers in them, a few groups of three would have no recoverers in them and a few would have three recoverers in them. In fact, of that hundred groups, no less than 27 groups would comprise three patients who all recovered. So your findings would occur by chance in 27 per cent of samples. Sadly, your experience of three patients getting better with the betel-juice-and-oil-of-squills remedy could simply be the way the chips fall; in fact, it is the way the chips fall 27 per cent of the time."

You are deeply depressed. "Never mind," the statistician tells you, "just go out and treat a lot more patients. If you treat 20 patients and *they* all get better, that result would happen by chance only one time in 30,000 million. If that's the result you get, then you *have* invented the cure for *digititis* and you *will* be a millionaire."

This is slightly better news, but it still leaves you with an important question unanswered. If something happens by chance 27 times in a hundred, nobody believes it. If an event could happen by chance only one time in a thousand, everybody believes it. So, where's the cut-off—what's the level at which the world will believe the results are real and not chance? "Well," the statistician replies, "funny you should ask that, but the whole international scientific community has agreed to accept the level of 5 per cent as acceptable. So if an event could have occurred by chance fewer than five times out of a hundred, then we are all prepared to believe it's a real effect. But that doesn't mean," adds the statistician, who can hear you getting excited, "that everything with a 'chance level' of 5 per cent is *definitely* true. It just means that the chance of it being a fluke is less than 5 per cent, and we'll accept it for the time being. So if, for instance, you read the results of 20 different experiments and each of those experiments has the same 'chance level' of 5 per cent, then in all probability *one* of those 20 experiments *is* a fluke and happened that way by chance alone. And you won't know which of the 20 it is. Which is why if a result is important, the experiments need to be repeated several times to make sure the effect *isn't* chance alone."

"Oh," you say, now feeling less hopeful than ever, "but what if the chance level is one in a hundred; is it a definitely and absolutely and totally true result then?" The statistician sighs patiently, "All that would mean is that the experiment has a 1 per cent chance of being a fluke—it still *could* be a fluke but the chance is only one in a hundred."

"Well, that's all right," you say, "I'll settle for that."

"It rather depends on what you're trying to prove," says the statistician. "If you have a blurred photograph of an animal with one horn and you say it's a unicorn, then you need to have *very* solid proof because there's no other evidence of the unicorn's existence—we haven't got any in zoos, we don't have fossil unicorns or unicorn droppings or cave paintings of unicorns. On the other hand, we've got lots of goats, and if you take hundreds of photographs of goats, you'll find that one time out of twenty a goat gets photographed sideways so you only see one horn. That means that if you have a photograph of a goat, there's a one-in-twenty chance that the photograph could look like a unicorn. And that puts the unicorn hypothesis in trouble. Goats are very common, and a single photo of a single-horned animal—with a one-in-twenty chance of it being a goat—is certainly not good enough proof by itself of the existence of a unicorn."

"Ah," you say and hurriedly shove the blurred photograph that you thought was a unicorn under a cushion, "but let's get back to my betel-juice remedy. Suppose I think it works some of the time but not all of the time. If the disease gets better in 33 per cent of cases by itself, but if I find let's say that half my patients get better—what then? Can I say I get a cure rate of 50 per cent with betel juice when the spontaneous recovery rate is 33 per cent? And how many patients will I need to make sure *that* that isn't a chance finding?"

You hear the statistician feeding the data into a computer. (Actually, that test is so simple that it's programmed into hand-held solar-powered credit-card-thin calculators that cost less than $20 and also tell you the time in 200 cities of the world, remind you of up to 80 birthdays and anniversaries and play "Waltzing Matilda" for no apparent reason when you're least expecting it.) The statistician has his answer. "If you want to prove your remedy genuinely cures 50 per cent of the patients, when the spontaneous recovery rate is 33 per cent," he says, "to prove that with a chance level of less than 5 per cent, you will need 140 patients."

"Thank you," you say, "I'll phone you in six months" and you put the telephone down, a wiser but sadder scientist than you were in the first moments of your eureka high.

Is conventional medicine a science?

It is a commonly held belief, particularly among conventional doctors, that most of conventional medical practice is based on good scientific evidence and fundamental biological principles. But how much is "most" in reality? Sadly, the answer is "Not very much." In fact, the best estimates[22] suggest that approximately 15 per cent of medical practice is based on sound science. In other words, 85 per cent of it isn't.

In short—and it's important to be honest about it—the process of attempted refutation has been applied only to a small proportion of medical practice. The balance is still untested and therefore—until proven otherwise—an assembly of accumulated clinical observations, folklore, fad, fashion, prejudice, old wives' tales, institutionalized phobia or prejudice and plain old hokum.

This is a most uncomfortable piece of data, and the discomfort that most conventional doctors feel may well account for the some-what defensive attitudes that are revealed by the challenge of complementary practitioners—particularly if those complementary practitioners claim that their techniques are based on sound scientific principles and solid evidence.

So is complementary medicine resting on better scientific foundations—or is the pot calling the kettle black?

Is complementary medicine a science?

Now we can look at the results of investigations into the effectiveness of various methods of complementary medicine—but with two caveats. First, as we've just seen, a trial is one method of finding out whether a particular treatment affects the course of a disease or illness. You need the results of a trial to back up a claim such as "Treatment X is better than antihistamines for hay fever" or "Treatment Y cures cancer in 75 per cent of cases." If the only claim for a treatment is "Thousands of people have taken the treatment and three-quarters of them *feel* better" then you don't need a trial, you need a simple survey. If 75 per cent of the people who try the therapy say they feel better, that's that, you've proved your claim. The whole point is that there are many things that make people feel better. It is only when a healer claims that a treatment is making a person *get* better, or that a complementary treatment is better than conventional methods, that a trial is needed. Second, we can examine here only the methods of complementary medicine in which some systematic investigations have been done. It is simply impossible to mention every form of complementary medicine—there are hundreds and the number is growing all the time. In the great majority of treatments, no systematic attempts have been made to evaluate the therapy and so there is insufficient information to say whether the treatment actually works.

In this section, therefore, we shall be looking at those types of complementary medicine for which there is some data, and we shall look at its validity—and that means that only a relatively small proportion of complementary medicine methods will be included here.

Controlled trials in complementary medicine

Compared to the great array of different therapies and the large number of different—and mutually exclusive—theories of human disease, there are not many well-designed and well-executed studies in complementary medicine. We have already mentioned some of the negative ones (for instance, in iridology), and a few miracle remedies, particularly in cancer, have been formally tested and found to be inactive (krebiozen and laetrile, for example). But a few studies have shown important results—and they are worth reviewing here.

Acupuncture: In many respects, acupuncture is the classic case of a complementary therapy that has been rigorously tested and proven to be effective and valid. Acupuncture analgaesia (and anaesthesia) is a reproducible and reliable phenomenon. For over 2500 years, Chinese patients have had all kinds of interventions—including surgery—while under acupuncture anaesthesia. This proves that something about acupuncture raises the patient's pain threshold during the procedure. The first reports and techniques of acupuncture anaesthesia came to Europe in the 1950s and to the United States after President Nixon established links with China in 1972. Initially, Western physicians found it difficult to accept the evidence supporting acupuncture because there was no consensus view on the mechanism by which it might work. Some scientists hypothesized that it could have been a cultural phenomenon related to the placebo effect, or perhaps hypnosis or even mass hysteria. Later, another hypothesis suggested that stimulation of the acupuncture meridians somehow altered the way in which pain messages were transmitted up the spinal cord.

With the discovery of endorphins, however, acupuncture suddenly became much more acceptable to conventional researchers and physicians. The fact that some—if not all—of acupuncture's effects can be abolished by naloxone suggested that acupuncture effects were mediated at least in part by endorphins.

However, an acceptable explanation of mechanism is only part of the story. The fact that a treatment *might* work by any given mechanism doesn't necessarily prove that it *does* work by that mechanism—or at all. Over the last few years, however, several studies have tested the hypothesis that acupuncture might work by placebo effect only and have compared true acupuncture (with needles placed on true meridian points) with sham acupuncture (with needles placed on points that are not part of any meridians). Trials such as these would be negative (i.e., both groups equal) if acupuncture worked only by a placebo effect. As it turns out, most of these trials are positive and show that acupuncture reduces acute pain significantly more effectively than sham acupuncture.[23] The exact role of acupuncture in clinical medicine—its use and its value in chronic pain and addiction, for example—is still undecided.[24] However, sufficient evidence from well-designed animal studies and from randomized controlled trials is available to demonstrate that acupuncture analgaesia is a real and reproducible phenomenon. As one author put it, "We know more about acupuncture analgaesia mechanisms than many conventional procedures. Perhaps the time has come to stop calling acupuncture an 'experimental procedure'."[25]

Chiropractic/osteopathy: There have been two major randomized trials of chiropractic manipulation for lower back pain, and they have both shown that chiropractic manipulations produce better relief of the back pain than treatment in a hospital orthopaedic department or by the family doctor.[26] These trials—well-designed, well-conducted and involving sufficient numbers of patients—should end the controversy about chiropractic medicine for *low back pain* but they don't prove anything else. They show—scientifically—that chiropractic manipulators are good at massage and manipulation. They don't prove that back pain is really caused by misalignment of the pelvis or vertebrae, and they don't prove—as some chiropractors claim—that *all* human disease is related to misalignment of the skeleton. All that one can state for certain is that if you have lower back pain, you'll probably do better at the chiropractor's than at your family doctor's or hospital orthopaedic department.

Reflexology: Reflexology is immensely popular, particularly in the United States, and it is popularly perceived to be as established and verified as osteopathy or acupuncture (with both of which reflexology has certain features in common). In fact, reflexology, unlike osteopathy, has little or no overlap with anything that conventional doctors do (apart perhaps from the incidental side effects of the chiropodist's craft).

The philosophy of reflexology is based on the hypothesis that connections exist between the foot and every other part of the body. In the same way in which iridologists believe that the body is represented in the iris, so reflexologists believe in the existence of ten channels that join parts of the foot with ten zones covering the rest of the body. These energy channels, it is believed, can become blocked and a reflexologist believes that she or he can feel minute lumps beneath the skin in certain areas of the foot representing the part of the body that is malfunctioning. With a specific type of foot massage, the reflexologist claims to be able to break up the crystals that are present in the lumps and that are then absorbed by the body's waste system and excreted through sweat or in the urine. Reflexologists use charts of the foot to help them locate blockages and relate them to parts of the body—generally speaking, the toe end of the foot represents the head, and the heel end the lower parts of the body. Reflexologists claim that the therapy works effectively for congestion of various types; one pamphlet describes its uses to "unblock sinuses, relieve migraine, assist the function of the pancreas and liven up a sluggish liver."

Adherents of reflexology claim that the technique can be traced back for 5000 years or more, but its documented use is very recent. Its rise in the modern era began in 1932 with the publication of *Stories the Feet Can Tell* by Mrs. Fred Stopfel. As with many other types of complementary medicine, there isn't any solid or reliable information to base an assessment on. One can certainly agree with reflexologists who state that the vast majority of their patients feel better after the therapy. One text says, "Most reflexologists report that many of their patients come simply because they find the treatment irresistible for dispelling symptoms of stress: they feel relaxed and calm after the session and go home to sleep like dogs."[27] It is gratifying—to patient and healer—that symptoms (particularly stress-related) are relieved by reflexology, but so far there is no published evidence of any proven improvement in objective tests such as those of pancreatic or liver function.

Traditional Chinese Medicine: There is one study of a particular form of complementary medicine that is so clear nobody could possibly dispute it—and it does point the way in which future trials of complementary medicine should be conducted and interpreted. The trial was conducted at the Great Ormond Street Hospital for Sick Children in London after a series of quite unusual cases were seen in which children with very bad eczema that was resistant to standard therapy suddenly improved. The conventional doctors who saw the first three or four cases like this asked what had happened. They were told the same thing—that the children had been seen by a Chinese doctor in a little crowded office round the corner and that he had been giving the children a traditional Chinese concoction of 12 herbs made into a tea.

Although it seemed unlikely that a herbal tea could benefit children with eczema, the doctors collaborated with the Chinese doctor and organized a beautifully designed trial.[28] They prepared a "sham" tea made of another set of traditional herbs that weren't part of the original recipe. Then they gave the correct tea or the sham tea (in randomized order) for eight weeks, separated by four weeks' "wash-out period"—half the patients getting the real tea followed by the sham tea, and the other half getting the reverse order.

The results were so dramatic that there can be no argument about them. As can be seen clearly from the graph on the following page, when the children took the real tea, their eczema improved dramatically; when they took the sham tea, it got dramatically worse.

This is the sort of trial that should be done for every type of therapy that claims impressive results. Of course, the clear-cut effectiveness of the real tea doesn't tell us why it works. It may be that one of the 12 herbs contains a chemical that is far more potent than any anti-itch medicine we have seen so far, or it may be that the combination of all the herbs has some effect on the manufacture of itch-transmitter in the skin or on chemicals made during inflammation. At present all we can see is that it works—and it works very well and with effects that cannot be argued with. It's worth bearing in mind results like these as we look at the results of similar trials in homeopathy.

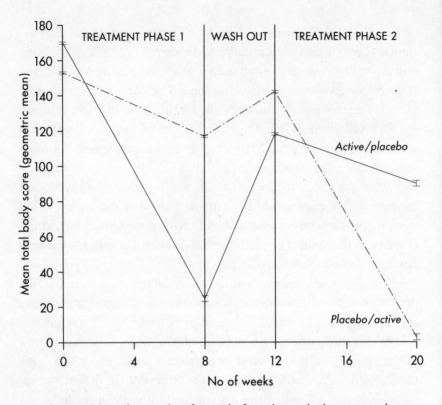

This figure shows the results of a trial of Traditional Chinese Medicine (TCM) herbal tea compared to a dummy (placebo) tea. The patients were children with severe eczema that had not improved on standard therapy, and they were randomly allocated to one of two groups. Half the children were given genuine TCM tea for two months followed by a one-month "wash-out," followed by sham TCM tea. The two groups show dramatic differences in the amount of skin reddening ("erythema") recorded by the doctors at each stage. When the patients who received the genuine tea first went on to receive the placebo tea, their eczema got much worse, and when the other group changed over from the placebo tea to the genuine TCM tea, their eczema improved dramatically over the two months. This result is clear and impressive.

Source: M.P. Sheehan and D.J. Atherton, "A controlled trial of traditional Chinese medicine plants in widespread non-exudative atopic eczema," British Journal of Dermatology, v. 126 (1992) pp. 179-184.

The vexed issue of homeopathy

Perhaps the biggest single scientific issue in the whole of complementary medicine is "How does homeopathy work?" We must stress the "how" of that question, because that is the issue that matters. The controversy over homeopathy has raged for decades and, like many debates in science, at various times has created more heat than light. But two points can be made without any doubt or prevarication: first, the vast majority of people who take homeopathic remedies are immensely satisfied and get relief of their symptoms, and second, there is genuine doubt over whether this is a true therapeutic effect or due to the placebo effect.

The centre of the debate is really the problem of the unicorn in the garden. If a mixture of alcohol and water dripped onto tablets at such weak concentrations that it contains no molecules of the original substance does affect the course of human disease, then this implies that the diluent (water with a little alcohol) has a memory and is capable of transmitting signals without the original substance being present. Now, if you have followed the account of the hypothetico-deductive model of science in this chapter, you will see that nobody can ever say, "It is simply not possible that water has a memory—it cannot possibly happen that way." The only statement a true scientist could honestly make is "If the water-memory hypothesis is correct, then we shall have to re-examine a very large number of the laws of physics and chemistry that we have accepted as valid hypotheses so far. It's not absolutely impossible, but since we'll need a major revision of much of our understanding of the physical universe, the evidence should be absolutely and totally convincing." And therein is the debate.

The problem is that the placebo effect is so powerful. As we've discussed above, patients respond to placebos in large numbers and with dramatic effects, even when they are told the medicine is a sugar-pill. Hence, in order to accept the homeopathic effect is a true phenomenon due to some alteration of the water, it is necessary to establish that the homeopathic effect is genuinely different from the placebo effect. That means that any test in which the result could be due to the placebo effect is valueless for this purpose—and that's where the debate gets hottest.

The fact of the matter is that a very large number of trials in homeopathy have been done and published, but only a few of them are so well designed that the placebo effect could not possibly account for the results. A recent review of 107 trials in homeopathy gave a marking system to the design of the trials and in particular commented on the "blinding" of the trials—in other words, the way in which doctors and patients were prevented from knowing whether the medicine was homeopathic or placebo.[29] This might sound like nit-picking, but it's actually the most important issue in the whole controversy. If the doctor or patient knows that one medicine is a placebo and the other is a homeopathic remedy, the results could easily be due to the placebo effects caused by the doctor being more enthusiastic about one treatment than the other. That is why, with homeopathy trials, an absolute and water-tight system of double-blinding is essential.

Some of the best designed studies showed no difference between homeopathy and placebo.[30] Of the studies that show homeopathic medicines to be effective, there are only a few that really stand up to scrutiny—a British trial of homeopathy in rheumatoid arthritis, an Italian trial of homeopathy in migraine and a Scottish trial of homeopathy in hay fever. All were well-conducted and—it has to be said clearly—there could have been no attempt at deliberate deception or dishonesty. All showed that the patients receiving homeopathic remedies did better than those receiving placebo. But on close scrutiny, two of the trials didn't quite do that.

In the Italian trial for patients with migraine,[31] homeopathic mixtures (selected from a fixed range of ingredients in a near-classical homeopathic manner) were compared with placebos for 60 patients. The patients receiving homeopathic remedies had dramatically better scores at the end of the assessment period of four months. In fact, the results were so dramatic they would suggest that homeopathy is the most powerful treatment for migraine yet tested. These findings are of considerable importance and need to be repeated.

An English study was set up to replicate the Italian study, but with even more stringent criteria and design. The English study[32] limited entry to patients whose headaches were closer to the classical definitions of migraine, and all aspects of the trial were tightly controlled. The patients were given a homeopathic prescription (selected on homeopathic principles from a repertoire of eight remedies, in a manner similar to the Italian migraine trial), and then the pharmacy gave them tablets in a coded box. Analysis was detailed and prolonged; in fact, five major measures of migraine were assessed for a total of three months. The trial was well conducted, the remedies were in line with homeopathic principles, placebo effects were rigorously excluded and the follow-up time (three months) was very reasonable. The trial was negative; there were no differences between placebo and homeopathic remedies. In some respects, this was a rigorous and detailed attempt to prove the dramatic results seen in the Italian study—and it did not confirm them.

Two other major studies are worth looking at. In the British trial of homeopathy in rheumatoid arthritis,[33] the patients were given their medicines by a doctor who knew whether she was handing out placebos or homeopathic remedies. She took no further part in the assessment of the patients, but the point is that she might well have responded differently to the patients and may have introduced precisely those kinds of differences that the trial should have excluded.

The only published trial that is absolutely water-tight from that point of view is the Glasgow study of Dr. David Taylor Reilly for patients with hay fever.[34] The design is flawless. The homeopath prescribed the remedy (although it was not individualized to the patient, but contained the same extracts of pollen for all patients, thus partly violating one basic guideline of homeopathy, but acceptable in the context of hay fever). The pharmacy then gave the patient a set of tablets that were coded but not identified in any other way; the tablets were either the homeopathic remedy or the placebo, and nobody knew which was which. The patients took the tablets for two weeks (after all patients had had a "run-in" period of placebo for one week). During the two weeks' treatment, half the patients were taking homeopathic remedies and the other half were taking placebo. After the two weeks of treatment, the patients were assessed for a further two weeks. Neither the doctors nor the patients could have had any inkling of what tablets were being given, so no placebo differences could have crept in.

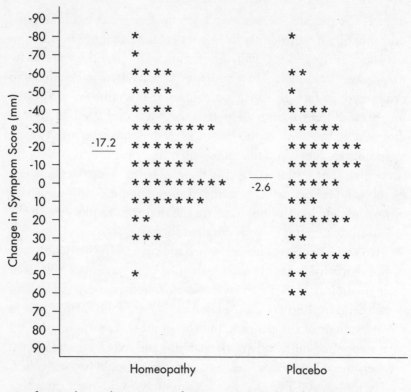

This figure shows the amount of improvement in hay-fever symptoms experienced by patients in a trial of genuine homeopathic tablets against dummy ones. The patients assessed how much their symptoms had changed at the end of five weeks, for two weeks of which they received either genuine homeopathic tablets or dummy tablets. Each dot represents the change in severity of symptoms that each patient experienced. The bigger the negative number the greater the improvement. The column on the left shows the scores of the patients who received the genuine tablets; the column on the right the scores of those who received dummies. Statistically, the patients who received genuine tablets fared better, though both groups had some patients whose hay fever got much better. In fact, the patients who did very well were divided almost equally between the "genuine" and "dummy" group.

Source: D.T. Reilly, M.A. Taylor, C. McSharry and T. Aitchison, "Is homeopathy a placebo response: controlled trial of homeopathic potency with pollen in hay-fever as a model, *The Lancet*, v. ii (1986), pp. 881-886.

The results showed that at five weeks, the patients receiving homeopathic remedies fared slightly better than those who got placebos. However, in the first week, the homeopathic patients on average did slightly worse. The homeopathic doctors' interpretation of this is that homeopathic remedies are known to cause worsening of symptoms followed by improvements, and this therefore confirms the activity of homeopathic medicine. But as we've seen from Freireich's plan above, this argument could be used to explain any possible combination of improvement, deterioration or stability. It's equally possible that fluctuations alone accounted for the differences. In Week 1, chance variations may have caused the placebo group to be better; in Week 5, chance variations may have caused the homeopathic group to be better.

The trial result has less than a one-in-twenty chance of being a fluke (and it is certainly rigorous and trustworthy) but the question is: Does it prove that the homeopathic effect is truly different from the placebo effect? Only an exact repetition of the trial (if it produces the same result and the same time course of deterioration followed by improvement) would prove that. This is why important trials of new remedies must be repeated before they are accepted as gospel.

Can one conclude that there is no such thing as a true homeopathic effect? Absolutely not—that conclusion cannot be drawn. A fair overview would say only that there is insufficient incontrovertible evidence that the homeopathic effect truly exists and that our understanding of physics and chemistry must be altered to accommodate the phenomenon. It is possible that future trials will dispel all doubts and that we shall have to undertake that revision and define the exact mechanism, but at the moment we don't have a clear photograph of a unicorn in the garden, and more trials should be done if we want firm evidence of the animal's presence.

However, if conventional science remains unconvinced about the existence of a true homeopathic effect, conventional doctors have a lot to learn from their homeopathic colleagues' interpersonal skills. In the course of our research, we interviewed and observed a dozen or so homeopathic doctors in action. To put it simply, most of them were excellent people-doctors and several of them were quite outstanding. The patient interviews with almost every homeopathic doctor whose clinical skills we observed were of such quality that they should be shown to every medical student as examples of How to Be a Real Doctor. The interviews had every single positive feature of effective doctor-patient communication—good body language and physical context, active listening, careful eliciting of the patient's problems, acknowledgement of the patient's experience, clear explanation of the diagnostic and treatment plan and clear statements of what would happen next.

In addition, they each were excellent conventional diagnosticians and had prevented potential disasters in the past by spotting serious illnesses (quite often when those diagnoses had been missed by other doctors). Furthermore, as counsellors and psychotherapists they each had considerable talent and intuition, coupled with great skill and experience. In one example that we observed in detail, a woman with a long-standing history of arthritis had her first consultation with the homeopathic doctor; she talked about her background and childhood experiences that she had never previously discussed with anyone. At the interview after the consultation, she appeared almost as a different woman—she looked physically and emotionally as if a great weight had been removed from her shoulders. And this was before the prescription for the homeopathic remedies had even been written, let alone administered.

In our view as authors of this book, we can see the merit of the scientific-sceptical viewpoint, which is that there is currently insufficient evidence to prove that homeopathic remedies are different from placebos. At the same time—and of far greater importance from the patients' point of view—it seems clear that homeopathic doctors are, on average, highly effective and empathic physicians, and that they meet their patients' needs in all senses of the word. However, that view would not necessarily please the homeopathic doctors themselves. Most homeopaths feel very strongly that homeopathic remedies *are* effective of themselves, and they would feel aggrieved at the suggestion that they are using placebos. (Perhaps that concern is justified—would anyone come to the Glasgow

Homeopathic Hospital if it changed its name to the Glasgow Placebo Hospital?). In that sense, therefore, the need to believe in the remedy may be an important part of the doctor's therapeutic equipment. Perhaps the homeopaths wouldn't be as effective if they knew the remedies themselves were inactive. It then becomes a difficult issue to decide whether scientific truth should be pursued even if it carries the potential for upsetting a useful and helpful therapeutic relationship between the homeopaths and their patients. Only society (the scientific, the medical and the patients' communities) can make that decision—and a consensus may take a long time to emerge. In the interim, however, while conventional science—appropriately—feels that the jury has not yet returned to decide the effect of the remedies, conventional doctors should start learning from the homeopaths immediately.

Another vexed issue: The Bristol Cancer Help Centre

No alternative medicine centre ever achieved as much front-page publicity (unwanted though it was by all concerned) as did the Bristol Cancer Help Centre in Britain. The controversy over the results of treatment at the Bristol centre was heated and damaging to all parties involved, and it may even have contributed to the tragic death by suicide of one of the main figures in the debate.[35] Because of the furor stirred up by the incident, it is actually very difficult—if not impossible—for any account of the events to be perceived as totally fair and dispassionate by both sides. Nevertheless, the story is extremely important and no book on alternative medicine could be complete without some mention of what happened. We shall therefore try to set out the main points in the controversy but will have to accept that partisans on both sides of the debate will accuse us of bias and prejudice.

The Bristol Cancer Help Centre was opened in autumn 1980 based on the experiences, philosophies and practices of Reverend Christopher Pilkington, his wife Pat, Penny Brohn (whose experiences and book *Gentle Giants* we discussed in Chapter 7) and Dr. Alec Forbes. From the time of the foundation of the centre onwards, the Bristol group emphasized personal wholeness, the value of psychological counselling and prayer and, in the early days, the Bristol Diet, which was predominantly a stringent whole-food and high-fibre diet supplemented by vitamins. Other therapies were also used, including laetrile. In their publications, the Bristol group consistently claimed that the combinations of therapies on offer at the centre

> do a great deal to improve the quality of life for every sufferer: they ease the pain, give more energy and slow the progression of growth. If they are followed completely and persistently they can, and do, save life.[36]

It was the claims that the therapies slowed the progression of disease and saved lives that caused the greatest difficulty with conventional doctors. After many discussions between the Bristol group and conventional doctors, a collaborative project was set up that initially reflected extremely well on both parties. The study, supported by the Imperial Cancer Research Fund, was to compare what happened to patients with breast cancer treated at the Bristol Centre with those with breast cancer treated by ordinary techniques over the same period of time at three conventional hospitals. The idea was relatively straightforward—the survival of the patients at the two types of centres (the Bristol and the conventional centres) would be compared as well as the quality of those patients' lives.

The study looked at 344 women enrolling for the first time with breast cancer at Bristol compared to 461 women selected as controls (matched for age and year of diagnosis) from the three conventional hospitals. To make sure that there was no bias against the Bristol patients, the data on any patient who relapsed within three months of first registering at the Bristol centre was taken out of the study and her results were not included. (This was to remove the possibility that patients who somehow knew or suspected that they were about to relapse went to Bristol, which would have the effect of making the Bristol group sicker as a whole than the control group.)

It was widely expected by conventional practitioners that the study would show no difference in survival. However, when the analysis of the results was published in the medical journal *The Lancet* in September 1990,[37] almost everybody was surprised. There were significant differences between the Bristol patients and the matched controls, and it seemed that the Bristol patients fared worse. The data showed the patients who had not previously had a relapse of their breast cancer were more likely to experience a relapse if they attended the Bristol centre than if they went to a conventional centre; for example, in the strictest comparison, of 126 patients who had no relapse when they came to Bristol, 21 patients suffered a relapse whereas only 6 of the matched 126 patients at the conventional hospitals did so. Worse still, the survival of patients *after* they developed relapses seemed to be worse at Bristol, the survival in the relapsed group at Bristol being 1.81 times worse than that of the control group.

The impact of this study was immediate and massive. The Bristol supporters pointed out—quite correctly—that the data had been published with haste and without all the review processes that might have been expected, particularly of contentious and controversial results. They also pointed out that the number of controls in the study was meant to be three times the number of the Bristol patients, whereas it was only 1.38 times the number and that the analysis of quality of life had not been published.

But perhaps the most serious questions were raised about the way the final figures were analyzed and about the differences between the two populations in terms of the initial tumours, local relapses of breast cancer (in the scar or in the lymph nodes in the armpit) and metastases (spread of the cancer to distant sites). The basic—and unresolved—issue was whether the differences between the Bristol patients and the conventional patients were enough to explain all the differences in outcome or not.

The authors of the study felt that they had eliminated the major sources of potential bias by excluding any relapses in the first three months (as mentioned above) through the use of a statistical method called the Cox regression analysis to correct for factors that are known to influence the outcome (such as size of tumour, number of lymph nodes involved and so on) and by using a "landmark" point of one year after entry to line up comparable groups evenly.

Despite these techniques, critics of the study felt that the two populations were still too different to allow accurate comparison; for instance, 86 per cent of the Bristol patients were younger than 55 years, compared with 73 per cent of controls—although there were no important differences in the stage of the tumour in the two groups.

The original authors worked over the data again and published an amended set of data that still showed the same overall results but with slightly altered figures[38]—the Bristol patients (excluding those with local recurrence) were 1.48 times as likely to develop distant metastases, those with local recurrences were 2.19 times as likely to develop distant recurrences and those with distant recurrences were 1.36 times as likely to die of them over the same time course as the controls.

There were recriminations, accusations and counter-accusations and apologies in many quarters. The head of the Imperial Cancer Research Fund felt that the initial differences were marked enough to enable only one conclusion to be drawn—namely, when patients know the outcome is poor, they are more likely to go to an alternative medicine centre.[39] It is now doubtful if any repetition of the study (which would be mandated in normal scientific circles) will be possible, although there are still hopes of a truly randomized trial.[40] Nevertheless, the study did show that once patients developed metastases from their breast cancer, they were more likely to die at the Bristol centre than at conventional centres; in other words, the Bristol centre had not substantiated its claim that its therapies prolonged life.

The results and the ensuing controversy are largely unresolved even now. An enquiry is underway at the Imperial Cancer Research Fund, prompted by charges of mismanagement brought by some supporters of the Bristol group. Nobody has a clear idea of why the Bristol patients seem to fare so badly, though some think that the Bristol diet might have been a contributory factor, and it currently receives far less emphasis at the Bristol centre than it did in the late 1980s.

IF IT MAKES ME FEEL BETTER, IS IT THERAPY?

Perhaps there is one important point that we need to stress before we leave the area of feeling better and getting better. Not everything that makes people feel better is necessarily therapy, but it's very easy for anything to sound (and even look) like therapy when the clients feel better as a result of it.

In North London, 45-year-old Rita Harris went to her hairdresser's. She had been treated for cancer of the ovary a few months previously, and the chemotherapy (with cis-platinum) had not affected her hair at all. But she felt terrible about it. "I don't know what it is but I just feel I *look* awful, and then that makes me *feel* awful," she said (quite loudly) to her hairdresser. He told her she looked fine (as did some of her friends in the shop) but carried on and did her hair. At the end of it, she felt wonderful. "I know you don't think there's a real difference," Rita said as she was leaving. "But I think there is, and that's what counts."

In the context of this book, that story seems quite remarkable for its unremarkableness. Of course, going to the hairdresser makes people feel better—that's why they go. But let's be very clear about something here: There are many services that people obtain that make them feel better, and not all of those services can legitimately claim the label "therapy." The hairdresser, for example, would never claim that he was giving a form of therapy. On the other hand, it would be easy for him to do so if he wanted. He would only need to change the title of his shop to Tricotherapy Treatment Centre and give his assistants crisp new white uniforms and start referring to them not as hairdressers but as "tricotherapists." He could then print a glossy brochure that highlights the value of a calming, welcoming environment that not only treats the clients (now called patients) like persons but gives them magazines to read, background music to relax them and coffee if they want it. He could add in a few hypotheses that suggest that having your hair done improves the functioning of the immune system and removes from the body toxins that have accumulated over the previous weeks in the shaft of the hairs. If challenged, the hairdresser/therapist could certainly point to the dramatic way in which his patients improve after their therapy and the way in which their perceptions of themselves have changed, resulting in different interactions with their friends and family.

Although we have deliberately chosen a rather frivolous example, the central point is a serious one. When does something deserve the title of therapy? About 15 years ago in Britain, a socially minded woman organized sexual encounters for people who were socially isolated (such as old people and people who were physically handicapped and couldn't get out of their homes easily). There was a public and rather acrimonious debate about whether this woman was providing "sexual therapy," as she claimed, or simply "sex," as the tabloid newspapers claimed.

In practice, there is no sharp dividing line. Most cases are quite easy to sort out—clearly radiotherapy given by a 25 megavolt linear accelerator deserves the title therapy. Equally clearly, a hamburger and french fries cannot legitimately claim to be "fast-food therapy." But in between those extremes, it can be very difficult to decide where the true frontier lies. Yet the dividing line does matter, and it matters most when any practitioner—conventional or complementary—says, "What I'm doing *must* be therapy—look, it works."

The fact that an intervention works doesn't necessarily prove the truth of its underlying philosophy. Our hairdresser in the example might say something like this: "My results speak for themselves. They prove that my theories about toxins in the hair shaft are correct. You can see the evidence for yourself. When I do my patients' hair, they all feel better." Clearly in this example, the patients/clients are feeling better. The hairdresser might well believe that this was due to the removal of toxins in the hair shaft, but his theory would require much more in the way of evidence before it could be proven; for instance, if the hairdresser were of a scientific train of mind, he might try to prove his toxin theory in three steps. First, he might try to show that there were toxins in the hair shaft—perhaps by extracting material from human hair and injecting them into animals or cells in culture and showing that they had harmful effects.

Second, he might try to demonstrate that people who had higher concentrations of these toxins in their hair felt worse than others who had less. And third, he might do a randomized trial comparing one type of hairdressing technique that did remove hair-shaft toxins (the haircutting-treatment arm of the trial) with another type of hairdressing that didn't remove toxins (the control arm of the study—perhaps an equally good-looking hair-do with a perm and colouring but without the toxin-removing cutting) to compensate for the placebo effect. All of this is quite a lot more work than simply claiming the theory is right because the treatment works.

There are several types of complementary medicine that undoubtedly make patients feel better but that can lay only very tentative claims to being therapy. One such example is aromatherapy. There is no doubt that patients feel better after being massaged with nice-smelling oils. However, aromatherapists claim that the exact selection of which oils to use is a major part of the therapy. They claim that essential oils must be used. The question is: Would the massage be just as good if they used any nice-smelling oils selected at random? Similarly, chiropractors often attribute musculoskeletal pain to misalignment of bones, particularly the pelvis and spine. Their interventions make patients feel better, but that does not necessarily prove that an apparent difference in length of one-quarter of an inch between the left leg and the right does actually make any difference or is the true cause of the pain.

MIND OVER MATTER

Now we must address a crucial issue—what are the limitations of the power of the mind over matter (in this case, the matter of the human body)? We've already seen that the mind (or to be accurate, the patient's perceptions, beliefs and expectations) can influence the severity of almost any physical symptom. We've also seen the evidence of that influence in the placebo effect and in the other ways in which a change in the state of mind can change physical symptoms. There is a multitude of examples, but some of the simplest include bereavement counselling, which often alters grieving; psychotherapy and psychiatric interventions, which can alter a wide range of physical symptoms associated with psychological or physical diseases; specific therapy that can get an addict off drugs, cigarettes or alcohol and so on. The question is this: If the mind can influence matter in these somewhat mundane but still valuable ways, what can't it do? Can the mind cure the body of multiple sclerosis, cancer, AIDS or heart disease? And if not, why not?

The problem is that there are many different ways of interpreting the phrase "mind over matter." Some people use it to imply that there is a mysterious and unmeasurable energy force that can be directed by the mind and that can reverse disease. Others use it to show that the mind can alter the impact of diseases (one example of which is the placebo effect). This is a case that illustrates the ambiguity of the mind–over–matter concept:

Janice Martin is the young legal secretary with chronic back pain whose story we introduced in Chapter 2. She had fallen from a window two and a half years ago and had broken her back. In confidential conversation after the session with the spiritual healer, Janice revealed some other aspects of the story that might have had a marked influence on the case.

The day of the accident was quite an unusual one. Janice had been living with a man for about seven years, but he had refused to divorce his wife. He and Janice had been trying to have a child together. On the day of the accident, Janice had just found out that she was pregnant. She went to tell her boyfriend, but before she could do that, he told her that he had made his wife pregnant and she had just had his child that morning. Janice had no idea that he was still having sexual relations with his wife and, as she put it, "I had a complete breakdown." She became totally uncontrollable, and after trying to fight with her boyfriend, she ran to the window and threw herself out of it. Janice's accident was an attempted suicide.

Janice was found by a passerby under the window and, devastated with the physical and psychological pain, she did not say what had happened. Even when admitted to the hospital, she still found herself unable to tell anyone that she had thrown herself out the window. As a result of her silence about it, her boyfriend was arrested by the police and charged with attempted murder. Charges were dropped when eventually Janice was able to tell the truth. Janice recovered in hospital but the pregnancy miscarried.

Janice had not worked since the incident. Now, two and a half years later, she was ready to resume work and came to see the spiritual healer.

At the end of the hour-long session with the spiritual healer, Janice said that she was experiencing her first pain-free moment for years. The spiritual healer claimed that her healing had done this by unlocking the forces of Janice's mind, aided by spiritual forces outside her body. But, at that time, the spiritual healer knew nothing about the events leading up to Janice's back injury. Does that make a difference? There are strong arguments for thinking that the circumstances of Janice's injury might have an important bearing on how we interpret the outcome of the healing session.

Let's think for a moment about the incident in conventional psychiatric and psychotherapeutic terms. Janice's attitude to her back injury must surely be surrounded by a great deal of anger and guilt. At the time of the incident, she was totally enraged by the betrayal and deception of her boyfriend. She may also have been extremely angry with herself for allowing herself to be duped for so long and for becoming pregnant by such a man. The rage and the self-anger may well have contributed to her motive in throwing herself from the window. After the accident, there would almost certainly have been deep guilt—about getting her boyfriend arrested, about not telling anyone what she had done to herself and about losing the baby.

After two and a half years of unemployment, a major operation, constant pain and dozens of different analgaesics, Janice said that she was now ready to begin again. In terms used by some psychotherapists, she was ready to "let go of her pain" and to forgive herself. It doesn't require the genius of a Dr. Freud to see that Janice might have been flagellating herself with her pain, punishing herself (and her boyfriend, directly and indirectly) for her gullibility, her rage and her injury to herself and the unborn child. Now, she was asking for forgiveness—and the session with the spiritual healer could easily have provided a socially and psychologically accept-able ritual of forgiveness. The healer said it wasn't Janice's fault; it was all due to the block in the energy field, and it could be fixed by a power beyond Janice's but still using the abilities of her own mind. Nothing could bring her more complete forgiveness, noth-ing could exonerate her of her burden of guilt and poor self-esteem as quickly and as perfectly.

Of course, this explanation, although logical and consistent with our understanding of psychotherapy, has not been proven. It is still possible that the healer did command some energy forces in Janice's spine to unblock. However, since all the facts of the case were not known to the healer, shouldn't we consider them before immedi-ately accepting Janice's improvement as evidence of the spiritual forces?

Janice's case may really be an example of mind over matter, but does it necessarily prove the existence of a healing force outside the conventional realm of psychotherapy? The more mundane psy-chotherapeutic meaning of "mind over matter" may be sufficient to explain the facts—although invoking different and unusual mys-tical forces may be much more attractive and acceptable to the patient and to the general public. However, there is one area in which this dispute has progressed from an academic matter or interpretation into a major schism of faith, and that is the issue of whether the human mind can change the course of cancer.

Yet another vexed issue: mind over cancer

The view that attitude of mind, and particularly optimism, can change the course of cancer has never been more popular. Perhaps the best evidence of this widespread and firmly held belief is the popularity and success of Dr. Bernie Siegel, whose books on hope and healing have sold millions of copies. (He refers to himself as Bernie—and asks everyone else to do the same—in order to dis-tance himself from the conventional authoritarian role of the doc-tor.) Bernie noted that cancer patients who did unexpectedly well had certain personality traits and characteristics in common. His books contain many anecdotes of patients who had very specific purposes in their lives and whose survival was longer than expected (often much longer) allowing them to fulfil those purposes. This has led him to believe strongly that a positive hopeful attitude and a sense of purpose can cause a prolongation of survival for someone with cancer. He believes that being loved and giving love are the main components of this process. His books (*Love, Medicine and Miracles*[41] and *Peace, Love and Healing*[42]) exhort people to understand, forgive and love themselves and to love other people. Of course, no sane person could possibly disagree with those recommendations; the only area of dispute is whether these changes in mental attitude and behaviour will cause a longer life. Bernie is quite certain that hope prolongs survival. When challenged, he is extremely honest and open about the lack of statistical evidence for this hypothesis and agrees that research into the effects of his own therapy group (the E-CaP group) did not in fact demonstrate any prolongation of life.[43] However, he cites as support of his idea a fascinating and important piece of research carried out by Dr. David Spiegel (we'll continue to use first names to avoid the confusion caused by the similar-sounding names) at Stanford Medical Center. In 1979, David Spiegel started a study to assess the impact of group therapy on the quality of life of patients with metastatic breast cancer. He wanted to see if group therapy (an hour and a half per week) plus monthly group therapy for the husbands plus additional techniques for pain control (which basically amounted to auto-hypnosis) would help the patients experience a greater quality of life.[44] The research compared patients who got this therapy with patients treated at the same medical centre by the same medical oncologists but without any additional group therapy. Interestingly, David Spiegel noted that the patients who received the weekly group therapy became involved with each other socially. They visited each other's houses, encouraged each other when there were medical problems, visited each other in hospital and supported each other at times of grief or bereavement. His original paper showed that all this activity did indeed improve the quality of the patients' lives. However, David Spiegel didn't expect this type of therapy to prolong survival, and when Bernie Siegel's hypothesis became widely believed, he went back to the medical records of the patients in the original study to see what happened to them. To his surprise, he found that the patients who had received the group therapy survived on average nearly 18 months longer than the control group.[45] His publication mentions specifically that at no point were any of his patients encouraged to believe that the group therapy would change their survival in any way (particularly since none of the workers believed that it would) and that patients in the group were encouraged to accept the probability of their own death. David Spiegel firmly maintains that his study does *not* show any effect of hope or optimism—rather it demonstrates the value of social networking and support. He maintains that the behavioural change produced by the therapy is probably an improvement in the patients' ability to cope with stress and cannot be adduced as evidence that hope prolongs survival. He feels that his results might be attributed to any (or all) of four causes: (a) "what your granny always told you"—that if you look after yourself properly (including good meals and exercise), you'll live longer; (b) that social support encouraged better use of medical facilities and greater co-operation with the doctors; (c) that better stress management changed the hormone balance of the patients, perhaps reducing levels of stress hormones; and (d) that the intervention improved immune function and changed the body's resistance—not in some mystical way related to visualization or attitude, but by means of humoral factors related to stress management.

CONCLUSION: HEALER AS DRUG

This issue of what it is that makes a patient better is really the essence of this whole book. It's so fundamental to the way in which patients and healers react to each other that it may be very difficult for either of them to see what is going on at the time.

In the last two chapters, we've been looking at some of the things that make it so difficult to tell why a patient is getting better—and in this chapter we've concentrated on the patient's expectations of the intervention (the placebo effect) and the impact of the healer himself or herself. As we've seen, we are dealing with very powerful effects.

We are talking about effects that are so powerful they can make Mrs. White feel that her arm is getting less swollen while it's actually getting bigger, they can make Peter Carol go to sleep in the middle of a heroin-withdrawal storm, they can cause dramatic improvements in dozens of patients' migraine while they're in a homeopathy trial, and there is almost no bodily symptom that they cannot improve in approximately one-third of cases. So why do we say "*just* the placebo effect"?

The word "just" should never have been allowed into this phrase. The medical profession would never have allowed it into the description of any other treatment; for example, most doctors would be enraged if anyone said, "Digitalis improved cardiac function in about a third of these cases—but that's *just* the digitalis effect." Or "Calmazepam cured the anxiety attacks in about one-third of cases, but that's *just* the calmazepam effect." If an intervention reduces symptoms in a third of cases, there is no "just" about it—it's important treatment and we need to learn how to use it.

It is quite possible that this is a major question that will need to be addressed by the medical profession as a whole. At the moment, healers—all healers, including both conventional doctors and complementary practitioners—feel somewhat uneasy about using a substance if they *know* it's a placebo and that its action on the patient's symptoms is somehow mediated by the patient's mind. Even though it has been shown that the power of a placebo is only slightly diminished if the doctor tells the patient it's a sugar-pill without action in the disease,[46] most doctors still feel that something isn't quite right about using them knowingly. Homeopathic doctors, for example, are usually quite adamant that they would have to give up using homeopathic remedies if it were ever proved definitively that they exerted their benefits only by placebo effects.

Which raises a major question: Why?

Why should a doctor or a healer feel inhibited about using a therapy that reduces symptoms in a third of cases and has no serious side effects at all? If the patients are not being deceived (for instance, if the doctor explains—as in the study cited above—that the drug is without action in that disease, but that a third of patients taking it will feel better), what is stopping us from using it? If everybody now accepts that people can feel ill without having an organic disease, why can't those people be given treatment that works without an organic effect? If a patient has flatulence and low back pain and investigations have shown that there is no serious disease process going on, what is wrong with fixing her symptoms with a medicine that has no organic action on any body process and no organic side effects?

The placebo may exert its effect by another method—that of bringing the doctor into closer contact with the patient. If the doctor believes in the therapy, he or she may feel much more comfortable with treating the patient and that comfort itself may bring secondary comfort to the patient. Perhaps, then, a homeopath's belief in homeopathic remedies and a crystal-therapist's belief in the energy of crystals and an aromatherapist's belief in the value of essential oils are all necessary to bring the healer close to the patient. Once close to the patient, the healer can use her or his intuitive abilities, such as counselling and empathizing, to their maximum effect. Perhaps the therapist even *needs* to believe in the remedy in order to be able to be a therapist or counsellor—and if so, that's fine. If it needs a few white pills or a group of crystals or a sweet-smelling oil to act as a catalyst for a therapeutic counselling and support session, then what could be wrong with that?

At its most basic level, it may be that the placebo effect is a reflection of man's fundamental desire for a magic therapy—we are so hopeful of a remedy that we imbue even an inactive remedy with magical powers. But the placebo effect also shows us something very plainly—if the patient believes in the magic, the magic works. If that does illustrate a fundamental feature of mankind's reactions to illness, then that's all right—but let's use it for the benefit of the patient and not ignore it. Of all the things that we can learn from the public's migration to complementary medicine, the placebo effect and the healer-as-drug effect are the most important lessons. To ignore them totally would be a terrible waste.

9. Synthesis: Magic and Medicine

Diseases need medicine, but human beings who suffer will always need a touch of magic.

In this final chapter, we have to make a confession. The title of this book is fraudulent. Magic or medicine is a false dilemma; in fact, it is not a dilemma at all. There is no necessity—nor any realistic possibility—of choosing between them. When human beings are ill, they require magic *and* medicine; both are essential components of almost every healer-patient contact.

To conclude, we are going to summarize the differences and the areas of potential conflict between conventional and complementary medicine and then show that the apparent demarcation dispute is almost academic. Each of the two schools of healing has a different territory, and there are many ways in which both can assist the patient without coming into direct competition.

Before we examine that frontier, however, there is an important issue that underlies all of mankind's attitudes to illness. Perhaps we can best put it as a question: Why does all of this matter *so much*? Why do humans have such strong feelings about their health, about their illnesses and about their healers?

The answer that we propose here is a curious one, and perhaps the best introduction to it is by way of an incident that profoundly influenced one of us (R.B.) and in which an important and universal facet of human behaviour became apparent.

Why All of This Matters So Much

When I was about eight years old, there was a front-page story about a tragic explosion at an ice rink in the United States during a show for children. A gas line exploded under a tier of seats and many children were killed outright and their bodies hurled onto the ice rink by the force of the blast. The newspaper reports said that there was total chaos, and amidst the wounded and frightened spectators, several tragedy-struck parents were seen wandering about the rink holding their dead or injured children. Some of the parents were dazedly saying, "It's part of the show—it has to be."

I have never forgotten that story or the sense of the unfeeling randomness with which life often seems to end. But the most important lesson (apparent even to me as a child) was that some things are too horrible to believe, and that even though rationally there can be no possible doubt about the death of your child in an accident, something in our nature prevents us from grasping the painful truth instantly. In a state of shock, our cerebral functions throw up some less painful explanation, however patently impossible it may be; we try to believe it and we usually succeed for a time. That incident made me realize that the desire to believe is one of the most powerful functions of the human mind. Human beings seem to need and to use that power in order to defend themselves against the insults and attacks of an apparently insensitive and random universe.

The situation is similar when illness strikes—as it often does—randomly and unfairly. Perhaps illness and failure of the body, particularly if life itself is threatened, is one of the most fundamental insults to the intellect of a human being. That life may be diminished, shortened or ended randomly without any relationship whatsoever to the worth, the virtue, the moral fibre or the goodness of that individual is intellectually repugnant to most people. So unacceptable is the idea of random catastrophe that we are ready to embrace almost any other explanation first.

Randomness is an abhorrent and painful concept to grapple with. It is as horrible as—and, as far as human beliefs, is probably identical with—vacuum and void. It is such a deep challenge to our idea of order, justice and equity that we seem prepared to believe almost anything rather than accept that random or arbitrary events may shorten our lives.[1] But the sad fact is that many major biological events are quite random. Certainly there are high-risk and low-risk situations—if you smoke, you increase your chances of lung cancer; if you eat lots of fibre, you may reduce your chance of getting bowel cancer, heart disease and (perhaps, slightly) breast cancer. But even so, many smokers will not get lung cancer, some high-fibre eaters will get bowel cancer and, sadly, there will always be accidents, most of which happen for reasons that we do not understand. Perhaps in a century's time we will know it all, or most of it. Perhaps we will discover that if you are born without the XYZ-oncogene in your chromosomes you can smoke as much as you like and you will not get lung cancer, whereas if your liver cells lack the ABC-ase enzyme, even moderate drinking will give you cirrhosis. At the moment, however, much of that is a closed book.

It is that aspect of the "closed book" coupled with our human revulsion of randomness that causes us to blame the patient for the disease. Mankind has a long history of searching for—and apparently finding—things that the patient has done wrong that have caused the disease. Tuberculosis was thought in the early decades of this century to be brought on (in people exposed to the TB bacterium) by artistic or aesthetic personalities. As a matter of fact, the condition of pulmonary TB was also called "phthisis" and there was a well-described "phthisical personality" which was basically the stereotype of the thin artist starving sensitively in a garret.[2] This was thought to be an important, perhaps essential factor—as well as the TB bacillus—in the aetiology of the disease before it was discovered that good living conditions and social improvements drastically reduced the number of victims.

Similarly, the Victorians believed that Down's syndrome (previously called "mongolism") in children was caused by the parents being intoxicated at the time of conception. Had that been true, it would suggest that perhaps 90 per cent of all children would have Down's syndrome.

Other examples include the more recent ascribing of personality defects to patients who develop colitis. The so-called "colitic personality" was defined as an over-obsessional fastidious person who somehow brought on—or contributed to the cause of—his or her own colitis. That has turned out to be completely false;

any person who has explosive diarrhoea with loss of blood and mucus every hour (or even more frequently) will very soon become justifiably terrified about faecal incontinence and obviously deeply worried about his or her physical state and bowel.

The current fashion of suggesting that personality traits are important in the case of cancer is just the most recent version of the ancient art of blaming the patient. One study—which has not proved to be repeatable—suggested that women with complete denial or major rage against their breast cancer did better than "hopeless/hapless" types or even than women who coped well. The extraordinary popularity of the ideas of Bernie Siegel attests to the acceptance of that idea. In describing the exceptional cancer patient—the E-CaPs whom we mentioned in Chapter 5—he suggests that a patient who has cancer holds the future in her or his own hands. Take the right attitude, make your desire to live strong enough and you will increase your chances of survival. This belief is very comforting if you are doing well and are free of recurrence ("I'm alive because I really want to be") but it is extremely damaging and guilt-inducing if you are not doing well and the disease is progressing ("I'm doing badly—perhaps that means that I didn't want to live enough"). So the pattern goes on and perhaps will always go on as long as human beings have to face illnesses and the threat of randomness.

This, then, is why illness matters so much to us. Failure of our bodies seems to be a reminder of the existence of random chance and its power to affect us, and we find it difficult to face that directly. The affront is too great, so our belief systems are spurred into action to protect us from the vacuum and the void. The size of the threat of random illness is met by the immense power of our ability to believe. Although that is a good thing because of the protection it offers human intellect and personality, it is also a confounding factor. The power to believe warps our ability to understand and accept facts—as witnessed at the ice-rink tragedy. This may be comforting in many circumstances (at the time of first facing unpleasant facts, for example), but it may later lead us astray and make us potential prey to exploitation.

Perhaps this also explains why both doctors and patients tend to behave the way they do. Many doctors seem to be cold and detached when they are dealing with patients who are facing serious illness or dying. Of course, there are many exceptions, particularly among doctors who are trained in palliative care, but it is quite common to find doctors who distance themselves from the human problems of their patient's death by being scientific, occupied in research, or even using black humour (which may be why medical school revues are so justly renowned for their wit and sharpness). Surely this all comes about because doctors, like all human beings, don't have a good way of facing up to random death. So they try to erect a wall between themselves and the dying patient—a division between Them (the dying) and Us (the doctors who are now different and perhaps therefore immortal). That wall allows the doctor some space, the chance of holding on to illusions of invulnerability and a reprieve from having to face his or her own mortality.

The same process may underlie a patient's desire to believe in almost anything that holds out a hope, however faint, of rescue. Hope also helps to build a wall ("I'm different from the others because I'm going to be rescued"). Hence the urge to invest faith and belief in anything that promises escape from the threat is a powerful one. This is why ill people are so vulnerable, and why it is relatively easy (particularly for the unscrupulous) to exploit that vulnerability.

In Defence of Truth

If the fear of random chance contributes to our fears of illness, then part of the antidote is support from our friends and family, but another valuable component of the remedy is truth. Although it is initially more difficult, it is usually better in the long run to be honest when events seem to be random. It is fairer to all concerned to confess that we (healers, doctors or well-wishers) do not know the answers, instead of inventing an explanation that makes us appear knowledgeable and helps us exploit the vulnerability and gullibility of the patient whose urge to believe is so high.

The truth is important because we can't make intelligent and informed decisions without it. Of course, the facts alone are not enough, but we need access to the facts before we make our choices. Even undisputed and established facts do not necessarily tell potential patients the whole story and are only part of the composite picture.

For instance, let us say a new therapy has been discovered for bowel cancer. Suppose the initial studies suggested that the new therapy improves the survival of a certain group of patients from 40 per cent to 50 per cent. Then a large-scale test was carried out with many more patients, and the results confirmed those initial figures. During that period of testing, the investigators also used a questionnaire to measure the extent of nausea or tiredness that the patients experienced while on the treatment. Let us say that 80 per cent of patients said that they were "moderately" nauseated and "extremely" tired. Those then are the facts. But for an individual patient, whether to take the treatment or not does not depend solely on the facts. He or she has to decide how much that high risk of nausea or tiredness matters. In other words, decisions (for doctors as well as patients) depend not simply on the facts—the outcomes of the interventions—but also on the "weight," the psychological and personal value that the individual places on those outcomes. It is certainly necessary to have the facts in order to know what the treatment has to offer.

Only the individual can make the decision based on the facts, and that decision-making process depends on personal values and emotions. The "worth" of a therapy is not, therefore, equal to its success rate; the worth of a treatment depends on the worth the patient attaches to both its benefits and its costs. Information does not abolish personal preference—it simply makes the choice an informed one. But it will always be a choice. If we know that tamoxifen might make breast cancer regress and that coffee enemas don't, we can still make our choice, and we might still decide to choose coffee enemas. Even if a complementary cancer centre seems to offer no improvement in survival and if the quality of life may even appear worse (as happened in one recent comparison between a conventional and a complementary cancer centre[3]), patients might still choose the complementary methods because the meaning of suffering might be different in such an environment. It is quite easy to imagine that someone might choose to endure even a little more discomfort or more prolonged nausea in a complementary clinic because the team at that clinic make the patient feel more significant as a person. The sum total of physical symptoms does not take away the person's right to choose. Nothing should ever do that, and nothing can.

Furthermore, the search for the medical facts of the situation does not (and should not) abolish hope. The human mind is particularly adept at preparing for the worst while hoping for the best. In practice, this is the normal way in which most patients cope with bad news. If a condition carries with it a 90 per cent chance of succumbing to the disease, a patient may acknowledge that as a fact while simultaneously hoping that he or she is among the fortunate 10 per cent. Facing and assessing the size of the threat does not rob humans of hope and fight; on the other hand, the disappointment after a broken promise of cure often does. In defending the principle of truth-telling in human illness, physicians can be, should be and often are emphatic, supportive and sensitive to their patient's situation. To be truthful respects the vulnerability of the patient, allowing him or her to make informed adult decisions; to offer false hope exploits that person's vulnerability and utilizes the deep urge to believe anything when threatened. Whether the healer is a conventional doctor or a complementary practitioner, it seems only fair and sensible that the support and care offered to the patient should come from a context of honesty and trust, and not from deception or exploitation.

THE NEED FOR SOME MAGIC WITH THE MEDICINE

So far we have seen the different starting points of conventional and complementary medicine; now we can examine the areas of potential conflict and look for methods of resolving those conflicts and combining the strengths and advantages of both schools. Those conflicts did produce personal reactions in almost every practitioner, whether a conventional doctor or a healer. This is the personal reaction one of us (R.B.):

By and large, the official bodies representing conventional medicine initially reacted defensively to the apparent challenge of complementary medicine. I must admit that my own attitude in the 1970s was also defensive and angry. Along with many of my colleagues, I thought that many complementary practitioners were claiming superior knowledge of major diseases and purporting to be able to treat those diseases when we conventional doctors could not. We all felt distinctly challenged, as if fighting for our right to treat patients. Added to that, several schools of complementary medicine presented theories that jarred with everything we knew about the physical world. It seemed to many of us that in order to accept what certain complementary practitioners were saying we would have to abandon every other fact and theory we had learned about the universe.

Time has changed the stance of both camps. Recently, complementary medicine practitioners have reduced the number and size of the claims of cure or effective treatment for the more serious diseases, and there has been a far greater emphasis on the patients' symptoms and on the value of the patient-healer interaction in itself. At the same time, we in conventional medicine have had to face the hard fact that, overall, we have not been very effective at understanding the human dimension of our patients' medical problems. We have also come to realize that—in family practice particularly—at least one-third and perhaps half of the visits are not occasioned by a medical problem at all, but originate from some difficulty in the patient's life style or emotional or social environment, which is brought to the doctor when there is no one else to turn to.

Over the last ten years or so, it has become increasingly clear that conventional doctors are good at dealing with diseases and complementary practitioners are good at dealing with people. And each school has a great deal to learn from the other.

The healer–patient relationship is a complex one and comprises many different ingredients. Truth is important, but alone is not enough; doctors cannot be cold, heartless, uninvolved scientists (unless perhaps their cure rate is 100 per cent, in which case their patients *may* not mind their doctor's attitude). Equally, compassion alone is not enough (patients need effective medicines if they can help—otherwise we are no further on than the public at mediaeval fairs watching the medicine men sell coloured water).

The evidence now seems clear that complementary practitioners can help patients with the human dimensions of their illnesses, and can do so very effectively. Conventional doctors are not as good at that—yet. Even when conventional physicians have all learned to do that, there will still be enough work to go round. The pot of human suffering is easily big enough to require the efforts of both camps.

So doctors must learn to look after human beings and must learn to be what their predecessors were: healers. At the same time, conventional medicine has to recognize—and respect—the value of complementary practitioners in ameliorating the patients' human distress. There need be no conflict, provided that both camps are honest about their limitations. Exaggerated or untenable claims for miracle cures or large efforts on serious diseases have so far damaged the credibility of complementary medicine as a whole. Detailed evidence of decrease in symptoms, on the other hand, has bolstered that scientific credibility and pointed to a true role for some types of complementary medicine.

Having established the potential synergy (and lack of territorial conflict) between conventional and complementary medicine, we can now put forward some practical options that may be of value in the future.

SOME PRACTICAL RECOMMENDATIONS

So where do we go from here? If we agree that complementary practitioners and conventional doctors each possess strengths (and weakness) that the other lacks, how can the patient get the benefits of both? Practical problems require practical solutions and we've divided our suggestions into three main categories.

1. Areas in which conventional doctors can improve Communication skills: Slowly and steadily, the subject of doctor-patient communication is growing in respectability, prominence and popularity. In fact, within the last two or three years, it has earned a rare accolade—if a doctor in the United States attends a recognized course in doctor-patient communication, his malpractice insurance premiums are reduced by 10 per cent. The meaning of this manoeuvre is clear. Medical insurance companies have a great deal of respect for the financial bottom line, and it has been proven that doctors who are good communicators are sued for malpractice less often. Hence, the insurance companies' subtle inducement to doctors to improve their communication skills.

Medical schools all over the world are gradually introducing the interpersonal skills of medicine into the curriculum. Research is being carried out in many countries. Different techniques of communication are being proposed and studied, and the effects of teaching have now been shown to be positive and durable. Medical students can be taught to become effective listeners, and the effects can be shown to help their patients and to be durable over the years.

Family practitioners can be taught—in a few hours—how to handle emotions and how to assist patients with problem solving, and it can be shown that this produces doctors who are actually better at diagnosing psychiatric illnesses (particularly depression) and that their patients have a higher recovery rate.[4]

In fact, conventional medicine is almost at the point of defining a universally accepted core curriculum of interpersonal skills, and (we can dream!) we may even see medical students having to take an exam in interpersonal skills. Perhaps one day, there will be a student who scores Grade A in Clinical Biochemistry and Histopathology, but has to retake his final exams because he (or she) got a Grade F in Empathy and Human Warmth. Perhaps.

The medical use of placebos: As we discussed in Chapter 7, placebos are extraordinary drugs. They seem to have some effect on almost every symptom known to mankind and work in at least a third of patients (usually) and sometimes up to 60 per cent. They have no serious side effects and cannot be given in overdose. In short, they hold the prize for the most adaptable, protean, effective, safe and cheap drugs in the world's pharmacopoeia. Not only that, but they've been around for centuries, so even their pedigree is impeccable.

In conventional medicine we frequently get into trouble using powerful and toxic drugs. That danger might be justifiable if we are trying to treat (or even cure) serious or crippling disease. The risk-benefit balance, however, is tipped dramatically if the original symptom is not severe while the side effects of the treatment are potentially life-threatening. Furthermore, many consultations with the doctor are prompted by a collection of symptoms for which there is no diagnosed organic illness. Surely it makes sense to look hard at the possible ways in which the placebo effect can be harnessed for the patient's (risk-free) benefit.

This is a thorny issue. It will require a great deal of discussion and, possibly, public debate. It may require far-reaching changes in the guidelines of medical practice, redrafting of treatment recommendations by the medical governing bodies and close supervision. However, whatever the outcome, the discussions themselves might make many constructive contributions to the analysis of our attitudes to disease and treatment.

2. Areas in which complementary practitioners might improve

If conventional doctors have to learn to become better people-doctors, then complementary practitioners should learn to become better scientists. In the vast majority of complementary practices, there have been few attempts to look carefully at what the remedy is achieving for the patient or what effect it is having on the illness. Of course much of this is awkward, and some of it involves a fair amount of work, but—as we noted when we talked about the coming of age of a science—it is the only way to demonstrate the truth of any claims. To carry on blithely making claims about curing illnesses and alleviating symptoms without any effort to show that those promises are being realized is unfair.

If practitioners of any form of complementary medicine would like to be taken seriously, they are going to have to do a little bit of work. That work has already been done in the field of acupuncture and—with less clear results—in homeopathy, but in the great majority of practices, nobody is interested in even finding out what proportion of patients actually feel better after the treatment.

More factual information would also help the serious complementary practitioners more than it would assist the smaller number of charlatans and outright frauds. Extravagant claims and fraud do more than rob the gullible customer; they cast a bad light on the entire field and cause even serious and worthwhile practitioners to be discredited. Some attempt to police any really extravagant claims would go a long way to increasing the credibility of those practices that are genuinely useful. This suggestion is not really revolutionary; every professional body has its regulatory body—conventional doctors have them, travel agents have them, real estate agents have them, plumbers have them. When the trade is in something as important as health, wouldn't a few visible attempts at establishing some minimum standards be welcome?

3. Ways in which patients might get the best of both worlds

Although it sounds hard to try and combine the benefits of both areas of medicine, there are actually quite a large number of different ways in which this might happen—and they each have different advantages (and a few disadvantages).

The free-market model: Complementary practitioners are absolutely everywhere. In many places, they are more numerous than conventional doctors. In Sante Fe, for example, a large city in New Mexico that's acknowledged as the U.S. centre of healing, there is an alternative practitioner for every 27 citizens, whereas there is only one conventional doctor per 200. This is free enterprise incarnate, and perhaps it's no coincidence that the name Santa Fe means "Holy Faith"—it does seem to be a city in which almost everybody is trying very hard to believe almost anything.

But Santa Fe is ahead of the rest of the world only in the degree of its free-market complementary health practices. The principle is the same in most parts of the world. Most countries have complementary practitioners who exist outside any regulations; they flourish as long as they are giving the customers what they want. In some countries (including the United States), health services are not free and are not regarded as an inalienable right of all citizens, and in many parts of the United States the complementary practitioners have the advantage that they are much cheaper than the conventional doctors. In some parts of the world, the complementary practitioners are the *only* healers—which certainly simplifies what might otherwise be a difficult choice for the consumer.

The "one-person-two-schools" model: In some areas, patients may be able to get the advantages of both conventional and complementary medicine from the same person. In Britain, there are several conventionally trained family practitioners who are trained in homeopathy and many more who are trained in acupuncture. There are practitioners such as Effie Chow in San Francisco who trained as a nurse in the conventional system but has a wide and long experience of traditional Chinese medicine and uses (or recommends) whatever modality she thinks will help the patient most.

The "one-building-two-schools" model: On the other hand, rather than have the two schools of medicine co-exist inside the same person, they could co-exist in the same building.

This is the model pioneered in Britain by Dr. Patrick Pietroni at the Marylebone Health Centre in central London. It is a group practice of approximately 35 people, including both conventionally trained family practitioners and complementary practitioners. The centre is now incorporated within the National Health Service (which means that it is free of charge to the patient at the time of usage). So far, this experiment in cohabitation and co-operation between conventional and complementary medicine has produced some fascinating results. Perhaps the most significant statistic is the considerable reduction in prescriptions. The average prescribing rate is 60 per cent less than the national average, and 36 per cent below the local London level. The average family practitioner in Britain prescribes approximately £85,000 worth of prescription drugs a year. At the Marylebone Centre, the figure per doctor is £39,000. The money saved on conventional drugs finances the employment of the complementary practitioners (such as the acupuncturist, osteopath, spiritual healer, and so on). And the savings are more than purely financial; the Marylebone Centre makes fewer referrals to the local orthopaedic specialists (because of their use of their own chiropractor) and far fewer referrals to the local psychiatric services (because of their own counselling and healing services). In addition to the savings, the patients seem to be very satisfied. (Further studies are being undertaken to quantify that impression.) As Dr. Pietroni points out, it is a major advantage for a family doctor who doesn't know how to help a patient with troublesome symptoms to be able to refer him or her to an acupuncturist or aromatherapist down the hall.

The Marylebone Centre demonstrates one possible way to combine the practices of the two schools of medicine and, as such, really deserves attention. It may well offer a useful model for the future.

In conventional hospitals: Complementary medicine now complements—in the true sense of that word—conventional medicine in several different acute care hospitals in many different countries. In the five major homeopathic hospitals in Britain, homeopathic remedies and diagnoses are available alongside conventional medical services.

In Liverpool, a fascinating experiment is being carried out on the Intensive Care Unit at the Royal Infirmary. It's been known for some time that life for a patient on most ICUs is unpleasant. Because the patients are always seriously ill, they are intensely monitored and treated. They may be on a ventilator (breathing machine) and unable to talk. They will almost always have intravenous infusions, often with additional tubes in the veins of the neck. They will usually have a catheter put into the bladder. The heart may be monitored; there may be additional tubes in the radial artery at the wrist and sometimes drains inserted into operation sites. On top of that, there is often the pain from the original injury or operation, and the muzzy twilight feeling that often accompanies analgaesics given for the pain.

And, even worse, because of the large number of things that have to be done to and with the patient, the friends and family are usually kept out of the unit for most of the time.

The typical ICU patient is ill, isolated, frightened and in pain, uncertainty and limbo. And yet most of that—if not all—is absolutely necessary if the patient is going to survive.

In the Liverpool ICU, Dr. Chris Wilkes and his nurses have started a brilliant experiment in common sense, humanity and decency. Realizing that the one thing the patients lack on the ICU is consistent human contact—part of the magic side of the patient's needs, perhaps—Dr. Wilkes and his nurses have introduced a program of aromatherapy onto the ward. Several of the nurses have trained in the use of various oils and massage techniques and give each patient several sessions a day.

The patients love it. And Dr. Wilkes makes no apology for a change that puts the human contact back into nursing practice on the ICU. Appropriately, Dr. Wilkes and the nursing team are now conducting a study comparing patients who receive aromatherapy to those who don't. Even more significantly, they may try to compare the use of the "correctly prescribed" essential oils with the other nice-smelling but "wrong" oils to see if the benefit comes from the massage or the oil. In any event, the results of those studies will be very interesting.

Another excellent example is in the Chinle Indian hospital in the Navajo Nation in New Mexico. The Navajo have a great number of significant traditions concerning childbirth, and these have been incorporated into the medical practices of the local hospital. In deference to local traditions, a large tapestry rope is hung above each bed in the labour ward so that the women can hold onto it during labour, there is an arrow on the ceiling pointing to the east (Navajo babies are meant to be born facing the direction of the rising sun) and although usually women in labour are not meant to be given anything by mouth (in case an emergency anaesthetic is needed), here they are allowed to take some traditional herbal remedies. And everybody is satisfied with the arrangements.

Who should pay

As we saw in Chapter 2, one of the most consistent features of all doctor-healer interactions is that the healer should be paid. In many societies, the healer simply collects directly from the patient. In other cultures, the government kindly interposes its body between the two parties, collecting from the patients before they become patients (i.e., health insurance) and paying the healer as the need arises.

When a society has decided—as a group—to pay for all or part of the medical services, does that society have an obligation to provide all medical services, conventional and complementary? In other words, for somebody who lives in Britain and gets all orthopaedic or gastroenterology services for free, does that person have a right to get aromatherapy or crystal healing or iridology for free if he or she wants it?

Although this sounds like a simple socio-political decision with the proponents of complementary medicine on one side and the medical establishment on the other, there are precedents for deciding this type of issue. Think, for example, of the use of over-the-counter preparations. If you get a cold, you might decide to go home from work early and have a rum toddy and go to bed. Or you might decide to call in at the drugstore and buy a bottle of aspirin or acetaminophen. Or perhaps a slow-release antihistamine preparation to dry your mucous membranes up. Or a nasal spray. Or all of them.

If the cold gets worse and you get a chest infection with green sputum and a slight fever, you might well go to your local doctor and you might expect a prescription for antibiotics.

The question is this: Who decides at what level the patient is entitled to receive treatment free? You pay for your own aspirin, rum toddy, decongestants and nasal sprays—but (if your government is that way inclined) you get your medical visits free. Why? The answer is: Because society has voted it that way. Our society gradually incorporates into what it calls conventional medicine those treatments that conform to certain patterns, require certain skills in their administration and have certain effects, and if it pays for medicines, it pays for the new medicines, too.

Perhaps complementary medicine can legitimately be compared to over-the-counter treatments. If you simply *want* a form of treatment, you go and buy it yourself. If you have medical need for it, it *should* be provided as part of the general provision of health care and should be subject to the same regulations and strictures that health providers have to comply with.

Who should be responsible?

Whether the individual pays for it or not, who bears the ultimate responsibility?

In the free market, the patient goes into the healer's shop and buys a remedy in exactly the same way in which he or she buys a pair of gloves or a garden hose. If it's what you want and you like it, you pay for it and you get it. The only difference between health services and all other consumer goods is that normally you can't take them back if they don't work (though you can usually sue the doctor or the hospital).

So whose responsibility is complementary medicine—and whose should it become? Obviously there is no right or wrong answer to this, but perhaps we can again use examples from what is already going on in self-medication. At present, a person with pneumonia (who has, let's say, a high fever, purulent green sputum and episodes of shivering) can ignore how ill he or she feels and go into a drugstore and buy some aspirin. The pharmacist may be well trained in the value of drugs in chest infections such as pneumonia, but if the patient simply buys aspirin, the pharmacist doesn't have any responsibility to recommend a medical opinion or a visit to the hospital. If on the other hand, the patient says, "I've got a pain in my chest, a fever of 40°C, green spit and shivering spells," the pharmacist is obliged to make a recommendation and not simply take a few dimes for the aspirin.

It would be possible to envisage a similar system for complementary medicine. If a person simply wants a particular type of complementary medicine and does not feel ill or think of him or herself as ill, he or she can pay for that healing in exactly the same way as a person buying aspirin. If the person feels ill and tells the complementary practitioner that, the complementary practitioner would be held responsible and liable if an important diagnosis is missed. If the person goes to a conventional doctor, it is up to the doctor to prescribe complementary medicine for free if the doctor feels that it is medically required, or to recommend a complementary medicine to be paid for by the patient if the doctor feels it might help but isn't medically necessary. In that way, the conventional doctor is the gatekeeper for complementary medicine for all patients who feel ill—and in that way patients with serious diseases are unlikely to bypass conventional medicine and be treated inappropriately with complementary medicine.

Obviously this is just a suggestion, but the approach is not new; it's based on the way the general public accepts some responsibility in drawing the line between self-medication and seeking medical advice. Were it to be implemented, it would require a great deal of discussion between representative bodies of complementary medicine and conventional medicine, and ultimately, public debate.

An Unanswered Question

Perhaps there is one question that we have only partly answered and that needs reiteration at the end of all this. Do the facts *really* matter that much? If the patients are happy with complementary medicine, do the medical facts really matter? Does it matter if the medicine is working or if the healer is effective or if the disease would have got better anyway? Does it matter that Brian Ledger thought homeopathy cured his mouth ulcers after 27 years when his story is typical of dozens of patients with recurrent mouth ulcers? Does it matter that a 57-year-old man thought his medicine cured his brain tumour, when he was actually recovering from a stroke? Does it matter that a man thinks his secondaries might have been held in check by prayer and a healthy life style when in fact he had asbestosis? Does it matter that a woman in her mid-forties thanked her acupuncturists for curing a bladder infection that she had never had? Does it matter that readers of *Gentle Giants* may believe that complementary medicine makes breast cancer shrink when it was probably the result of conventional tamoxifen? Does any of this matter that much?

The answer is: no and yes. No, it doesn't matter to the patient, but yes, it matters to other people and to anyone who wants to know the truth. For many thousands of patients, the healer-plus-homeopathy combination works and they are free of their low back pain, tiredness and flatulence (symptoms that conventional medicine is notoriously bad at fixing). For patients with hay fever or mouth ulcers, complementary medicine makes them feel better. For any patient with any symptom, the feelings are all the proof anyone needs; it doesn't matter what the treatment is or how it works as long as it works.

But with more serious diseases, the facts do matter. It does matter whether that 57-year-old man had a tumour or a stroke, because if homeopathy doesn't cure brain tumours then other patients shouldn't consider it as an active treatment option if they have brain tumours. If the Bristol Diet doesn't work, then breast cancer patients should be told that, so that they can stop feeling guilty for not following it. If Jim Collins did not have secondaries in his lungs, then nobody should be told that a new life style and prayer might make tumours regress if *they* ever have lung secondaries. If Penny Brohn was taking conventional anti-cancer treatment for six years in addition to her homeopathic, herbal, dietary treatments and coffee enemas, and if she didn't say clearly that she had been doing that, then that's wrong. If Maurice Cerullo tells seven-year-old Natalia Barned in front of thousands of people that she is cured of her bone cancers and she isn't, then that is wrong, and those thousands of people have been misled. These are examples of errors—either accidental or deliberate—but there are other instances and other ways in which damage can result.

But Surely it Can't Do Any Harm?

When a patient asks, "Can complementary medicine actually do me any damage?" the answer should be "Almost never." But there are a few exceptions.

As we've seen in Chapter 6, most complementary medicines

are remarkably free of severe side effects and toxicity. Of course, this may be related to the generalization that most of them also lack any direct effects on the disease process, but even so the benign and non-toxic nature of complementary remedies is a big selling feature. In fact, the safety of complementary remedies has led to a widespread impression that none of them ever cause serious problems at all. As a general rule, that's quite correct. The vast majority of complementary remedies are harmless, which contrasts them sharply with most of the powerful conventional drugs and interventions that carry hazards of varying degrees and frequency. But there are exceptions to all generalizations, and it's worth spending a little effort in looking at some of those exceptions.

By and large, complementary medicines cause problems in two ways—by acts of commission and by acts of omission. In other words, on some occasions (although they're very rare) the complementary remedy produces a direct toxic effect and does the patient some harm, and on other occasions (probably a little commoner) the harm comes from the fact that the patient neglects conventional treatment and suffers damage from a treatable or curable disease.

Acts of commission

As we've said, by and large conventional remedies are far more hazardous than complementary ones, but even so, occasionally complementary remedies do create problems, and this may be due partly to the common perception that they are absolutely safe and because they are "natural"—can't hurt the patient under any circumstances.

Perhaps one of the strangest forms of complementary medicine is the once-fashionable practice of giving coffee by enema. Several practitioners have claimed to have invented this, but the coffee enema became part of the treatment regime at Josef Issels's clinic in Bavaria and at Dr. Ernesto Contreras's laetrile clinic in Mexico.

The idea behind the coffee enema is bizarre and totally without any factual foundation. Most complementary practitioners regard coffee (by mouth) as a potential poison, full of toxic substances with dangerous effects on the pulse rate, blood pressure, fatty acid metabolism, heart conduction and so on. This is all correct, and it's part of the reason that those of us who are addicted to drinking coffee enjoy it so much. However, the bizarre part begins when the complementary practitioners start talking about what happens when coffee is instilled into the rectum. They claim that somehow the lining of the rectum does not absorb the toxins, and that in fact the exact opposite occurs: the coffee given by the rectal route actually *removes* toxins from the blood.

Sadly, they are completely wrong. In every instance known to us, the absorption of materials from the rectal lining is the same as— and in some circumstances better than—by mouth. For instance, almost every drug that can be given by mouth could be given by suppository; in some circumstances it's even more effective. In migraine, for instance, the patient often has poor absorption for drugs by mouth because the stomach's motility is badly affected by the migraine. During the attack, however, ergotamine suppositories work extremely well, because the rectal lining is not disturbed by the migraine. The same is true of dozens of other drugs, including anti-nauseants, bronchodilators, analgaesics (including morphine) and anti-inflammatories. In fact, the rectum is so good at the act of absorbing materials including water and electrolytes that in emergencies it can be used to rehydrate a patient who has become dehydrated from persistent vomiting.

This became very clear when two deaths were reported from coffee enemas.[5] The fatalities occurred in patients who had been given many coffee enemas over a relatively short time (either three or four per day or up to twelve a day). The fact of the matter is that coffee enemas can seriously disturb the body's biochemistry. The rectum is so good at absorbing materials that it absorbs a large volume of fluid into the circulation, which can drastically lower the blood levels of sodium, potassium and chloride. These electrolyte imbalances can be enough to kill the patient.

These deaths were from side effects of complementary treatment, side effects that probably would have been foreseen by conventional doctors; the outcome was not a specific side effect of the coffee as such, but was due to the complementary practitioners' not realizing the basic principles of human physiology and trusting that the body—or nature—could cope with anything, including fluid overload and salt imbalances.

Sometimes however—and again this is a rare occurrence—the complementary remedy itself causes a toxic reaction. Stories like this are relatively uncommon, although they probably occur a bit more often than they are reported in the newspapers.

> Ruth Conrad originally visited a naturopath for her arthritis. While she was there, the healer noticed a mark on her nose and said that it was cancer. He offered to treat it with some black ointment costing $10 and containing zinc fluoride (which is often used to strip varnish from furniture and in high concentrations is harsher than oven cleaner). She put it on her face every day for five days but the pain became so intense that she had to go to hospital, where doctors immediately operated on her. The effect of the ointment was so serious that she lost her nose, both cheeks and her upper lip and has had to pay $200,000 for 17 operations. When initially told of Ms. Conrad's intention to seek conventional medical treatment, the healer became angry and said that if he had known she was going to seek a second opinion, he wouldn't have treated her in the first place.

This was a direct effect of what was clearly a toxic therapy, but there is another group of problems arising from complementary remedies caused by the lack of quality control. Whether this is accidental or negligent will probably never be known—perhaps the manufacturers of some of the remedies just don't care about quality control, or perhaps they simply believe that because their remedies are natural and healing, they cannot contain anything hazardous. Nevertheless, there are some reported incidents.

> In Freeport in the Bahamas, a well-known alternative medicine practitioner called Lawrence Burton had been administering what he termed immunoaugmentative therapy since 1977 to over 3000 patients, mostly American patients with cancer. However in 1984, analysis of materials submitted by the family of a deceased patient revealed that the sera administered to the patient were mostly albumen, and all were

devoid of the components described by Burton as being essential to activity against the cancers.

Moreover, materials given to five other patients were uniformly contaminated with quite dangerous bacteria (including *Pseudomonas, Corynebacterium* and *Staphylococcus Bacillus* among others). Of even graver significance was the fact that four patients' materials were positive for hepatitis B[6] (the most dangerous type of viral hepatitis), and indeed two patients who received the immunoaugmentative therapy later developed hepatitis B when no other risk factors were present.

There was worse to come. In 1985, two laboratories in Washington and subsequently the Centre for Disease Control in Atlanta demonstrated particles of the HIV virus (the probable cause of AIDS) in samples of the serum given to patients.[7] The serum being given to patients to cure their AIDS or slow it down was actually capable of causing it. In July of 1985, the clinic was ordered to be closed.

While we're on the subject of damage caused by the unintentional inclusion of substances that accompany the remedy, there is something else usually regarded as harmless but that can occasionally produce severe problems—hope.

Hope as enemy

"A good doctor must never rob a patient of all hope" is a well-known adage, but unfortunately, it does not mean that hope is a totally non-toxic factor that cannot produce any side-effects even in overdose.

Marjorie Hagensen was a 55-year-old woman with breast cancer that had spread with secondaries in the liver. At the time these were first diagnosed, Marjorie felt quite well in herself and tolerated the initial chemotherapy with few side effects. After six months of chemotherapy, the liver secondaries were much smaller (as seen on the ultrasound scan) and therapy was stopped. Marjorie had heard of an alternative-medicine practitioner in the same city and went to see him. She did not return to her original clinic until a year later. By that time, she was seriously ill. She was jaundiced, her liver was enlarged, she had lost a great deal of weight and she looked thin and wasted.

She was in considerable pain from the distended liver. However, she was also very angry. In fact, she spent most of her time enraged with the alternative-medicine practitioner because he had been telling her for the last four or five months that everything was going well and that she would recover. During this time, he had continued to give her his alternative remedies while she became iller and iller. As it happened, Marjorie was very brave about physical pain and about the prospect of dying; what insulted her and enraged her was that she had been fed on a diet of false hope and patronizing encouragement. Had she been told the truth earlier on, she would undoubtedly have stopped treatment and spent the last few months of her life visiting her friends and family. She died deeply disappointed and extremely angry with the practitioner who had lied to her.

The situation is even more hazardous for those who believe strongly in the mind-over-cancer doctrine; holding out false hope—particularly if it relates to the patient's own personality and attitude—can induce deep feelings of guilt if the condition continues to get worse.

One patient with cancer went to the Bristol Cancer Help Centre to investigate the possibility of some kind of symptom control for her disease, which was no longer responding to chemotherapy. Her husband, an NHS administrator, wrote movingly after her death of one aspect of the Bristol approach. He describes his wife's account of a solo meeting with one of the therapists:

> The discussion went like this: "Why do you have cancer?" "I don't know; no one knows." "Ah, but where did it start?" "The ovaries." "Ovaries: what does that suggest? Eggs, life, creativity. Have you been denying your creativity?" We were amused by this idea until its implication sank in: you are responsible for your own disease. I see this as a thoughtless intrusion into a woman's life at a time when it was running out....
>
> We discussed the Bristol experience a number of times before her death. On the positive side there was a real concern for the individual and his or her needs in coping with the overwhelming fact of cancer.... On the other hand we were worried by the claims of success

that Bristol workers advanced but never substantiated (at least not to us), and by the underlying assumption that cancer patients were responsible for their own condition.

It is unnecessarily cruel to tell people they may be dying because they have failed to live, love, work, relax, or eat properly, whatever "properly" means. We might be able to do these things better, but what right does anyone have to say that these factors might kill us?

Where is the evidence?[8]

Where the mind-over-cancer doctrine is most public, the effects on the patient can be very difficult to alleviate.

Caroline Dixon was a woman of 37 who developed an aggressive breast cancer. She received standard chemotherapy after the operation, but 18 months later she developed a secondary tumour in a rib. She came to the clinic holding (very prominently) Bernie Siegel's book *Love, Medicine and Miracles*. She was in deep distress and spent most of an hour crying because she felt that the secondary tumour was a sign she didn't have the right attitude. "Bernie Siegel implies that if you want to live strongly enough, you'll do fine," she said. "Maybe this means that I don't really want to live and maybe subconsciously I want to die and abandon my husband and children." Her sense of guilt and personal failure were very deep, and it required many sessions of counselling to relieve her misery. In fact, her tumour responded to hormone therapy and she was then given radiotherapy to the ovaries (to alter her hormone balance) which produced a very long-lasting remission. The guilt was actually more difficult to treat than the cancer, but it did eventually disappear, and she stopped reading books about the effects of the mind over cancer.

Sometimes the hope that is given by the complementary practitioner can fly in the face of all reason and may cause great distress at the end of a patient's life. The following story is again an example from the practice of one of the authors (R.B.):

Helena Ross was the woman whose story we recounted in Chapter 2—she had cancer of the ovary and went to Athens (actually to see Dr. Alivizatos) after her cancer recurred and did not respond to chemotherapy. While she was in Athens, she received Dr. Alivizatos's regimen, including serum injections. At the completion of her treatment, she was told not to have any X-rays or ultrasound scans for several weeks.

She returned to Toronto and within a few days her abdomen began to swell dramatically. The clinical examination suggested strongly that this was due to build-up of fluid in the abdomen (ascites), a very common effect of recurrent ovarian cancer. By complete coincidence, Dr. Alivizatos happened to be visiting Toronto, and by dint of great effort and persistence, Helena's husband, Leonard, managed to speak to him on the telephone. He told him of the abdominal swelling and that the medical team suspected this was due to recurrence cancer causing the fluid.

Dr. Alivizatos told Mr. Ross there might well be fluid in the abdomen but if it was examined under the microscope, it would turn out that there was no cancer in it. Dr. Alivizatos was quite convinced that his treatment had helped Helena and that she was currently clear of cancer. Leonard Ross rang me in tremendous excitement and asked me to take a specimen of the fluid to test Dr. Alivizatos's opinion. I took a specimen of the fluid the following day, and under the microscope it was—exactly as I had expected—full of cancer cells. Helena Ross herself did not want to know the results (though she must have guessed it) but her husband took me aside to ask for the results. When I showed him the cytology report, he was crushed. His hopes had been dramatically raised by Dr. Alivizatos's misinterpretation of the situation, and now he was devastated.

There are several "what if?" questions that should be asked here. What if the Rosses had not been near a medical centre and simply accepted the view that she was cured (despite the fluid build-up)? Wouldn't they have been left with the impression that the Greek serum worked? And what if a specimen of the fluid had not been taken and tested? And what if somebody had done an X-ray or ultrasound, thus breaking Dr. Alivizatos's rule? Would it not have been possible for Dr. Alivizatos to claim that he had cured the patient, but that the conventional doctors had destroyed the benefit by disobeying his instructions?

With treatment like this secret serum, it is relatively easy to conceal or camouflage failure so that the patients and relatives firmly believe the treatment has worked—or would have worked if it hadn't been for somebody else's heavy-handed intervention. In this particular case, we obeyed the complementary practitioner's rules and proved that, in this case at least, his claims of success were false.

However, we must be even-handed. Hope is a powerful medicine, and it needs to be stressed that simply because hope is dangerous in overdose, nobody has the automatic right to destroy all hope for the patient or to force pessimism onto him or her. As has often been said, the human mind is quite capable of preparing for the worst while hoping for the best—hope and future planning are not mutually exclusive. It may require sensitivity and expertise for the healer to support the patient when hope of cure is fading, but it can be done,[9] and it is worth doing. As we've said at the beginning of this chapter, nobody has the right to remove all hope, but that is not, in itself, an excuse for telling the patient any old lies.

Acts of omission

Most complementary practitioners are very keen to say that they regard their remedies as a genuine complement to conventional medicine and not as an alternative to it. However, a few practitioners still do genuinely believe that their remedies can replace conventional remedies altogether. In many cases, this doesn't matter all that much. If somebody wants to stop taking aspirin for their headaches or antihistamines for their hay fever and puts their faith in an alternative remedy, then no serious harm is done. Sometimes, however, a serious condition that might be curable with conventional treatment goes untreated and may even cause death.

> Frank Glendover was a man in his early forties who came to his oncologist in Toronto with a lump in his left testicle. A biopsy had shown that the lump was a form of cancer called a seminoma, and his oncologist had done scans that showed there was some spread to the lymph nodes. The oncologist was quite sure that chemotherapy was the correct treatment and she discussed it in detail with Frank.

Frank was a naturopath—in fact, he was a member of the local naturopathic college, and he refused chemotherapy point-blank. After further discussion, he agreed to allow the oncologist to give him some radiotherapy, although, as she explained clearly to him, there was a far greater chance of the disease recurring after radiotherapy than there would have been with chemotherapy in his particular case.

Nevertheless, Frank remained adamant and the oncologist gave the radiotherapy. Sadly, the disease relapsed a few months later. Again Frank refused chemotherapy (which could possibly have saved his life at that stage). In desperation, Frank's mother rang the oncologist and pleaded, but legally and ethically there was nothing the oncologist could do. Frank was a mentally competent adult and if he refused therapy, the oncologist would be acting illegally to even attempt to give it. Frank deteriorated and died while still believing that his own naturopathic remedies would somehow cure him eventually.

Cases like this are fairly rare. However, even in the clinical experience of one of the authors (R.B.) there have been two similar cases—both patients with Hodgkin's disease. In one case, a young man suddenly stopped chemotherapy in the middle of treatment and went to the Bahamas for alternative therapy. He eventually returned to the cancer centre, by which time the Hodgkin's disease had recurred and was resistant to therapy, later causing the young man's death. In the other case, another young man came under great pressure from an alternative therapy centre in London to stop chemotherapy and go on a macrobiotic hypervitamin diet. He reported this to his medical team and was visibly distressed by the pressure. In the end, he persisted with his standard chemotherapy and went into complete remission, but less hardy individuals could easily have been persuaded to stop standard therapy under the bullying pressure at the alternative centre.

Of course, most respectable complementary centres would condemn behaviour such as this and insist that patients continue with their standard conventional therapy while they are taking any additional complementary therapy. Nevertheless, there are occasional complementary practitioners who do take this "either-or" attitude and for the curable serious diseases, sooner or later they will bring about someone's death.

The situation is even more serious when it comes to the care of children. Western societies consider that parents have a moral and legal responsibility to protect the health and lives of their children whenever that is possible, and cases in which parents had failed to do this because of a belief in alternative medicine are quite horrifying.

> Lorie Atikian died at the age of 17 months because her parents sincerely believed in the power of a strange variant of herbalism. The parents, Sonia and Khochadour Atikian, refused to let their daughter have routine immunization shots, which they believed would poison her. Instead they trusted her health to a herbalist, Gerhard Hanswile, who practised an unusual mixture of herbalism and mysticism. At the trial of the Atikians for failing to keep the child alive, Hanswile said that his health system was "hard to put in a nutshell" but that it was "based on the different planets...herbs are under different planets...Mercury for example was for stomach ailments." It was reported that part of Lorie's treatment involved her being wrapped in cabbage leaves. Right to the end of Lorie's life, her parents were convinced that she would recover. So strong was this belief that her parents could not see what was so obvious to outsiders, that Lorie was dying of malnutrition. Her body was so emaciated and wasted that when one of the ambulance attendants saw her, he testified that "I thought somebody had handed me a doll...I couldn't believe this was a human being."

Cases like this one are extremely rare, but they do illustrate—tragically—the immense power of belief that can delude parents into misperceiving imminent disaster.

Very few forms of alternative medicine would condone this form of behaviour, but there is one that does. It is called Christian Science and in the last few years, tragic cases similar to Lorie's have been coming to light and the parents have been indicted.

Christian Science was founded in the United States at the end of the last century by Mary Baker Eddy as the First Church of Christ Scientist. It now has approximately 3000 churches over the world and it is the largest single group that practises spiritual healing.

The problem is that the Church of Christ Scientist specifically proscribes conventional medicine. It regards all diseases as "discords of the body" and believes that God can and should cure them. "God is good and everything he makes is good. We believe we can challenge it [disease] and cast it out through prayer." There are now many cases in which this dogma has caused the death of children.

One of the most vehement enemies of this lethal doctrine is Rita Swann, who was previously a Christian Scientist herself. Then her son Matthew developed bacterial meningitis at the age of 11 months. Despite the obviously deteriorating condition of Matthew, Rita was expressly forbidden by members of the church to allow conventional treatment (which cures bacterial meningitis in nearly all cases). By the time she realized how desperate Matthew's state was, it was too late and he died.

Several other cases have come to light over the last few years. John and Katherine King in Arizona neglected the treatment of their 12-year-old daughter Elizabeth when she developed a cancer of the leg (a disease curable in about 50 per cent of cases). The tumour grew to a vast size and caused her death. Christine and William Hermanson were convicted of third-degree murder for allowing their seven-year-old daughter Amy to die of diabetes. David and Ginger Twitchell were found guilty of manslaughter for allowing their two-year-old son Robyn to die of bowel obstruction. That particular case was brought to trial in Boston, ironically the home of the founding of the First Church of Christ Scientist. In all, approximately 28 cases have been brought against parents in these circumstances, and in most the parents have been found guilty.

Obviously, there can be stupidity and negligence in any society or culture. What is so disturbing about these instances, though, is that this is not individual negligence or lack of common sense—this is institutionalized doctrine that causes death. The Christian Science church believes something that is manifestly false—that spiritual healing will reverse serious organic diseases—and the followers accept that doctrine even to the extent of over-riding their own parental instincts. While of course these cases are a stunning indictment of the gullibility of some parents, they are also an ominous demonstration of the power of human belief and its ability to alter perception even of the most obvious emergencies.

Cases like these are extremely rare and the point of detailing them here is not to raise hackles or cause widespread alarm. In the great majority of instances, complementary medicines are far safer and less toxic than conventional medicines, and even if they do cause the occasional serious injury or death, they do so far more rarely than in conventional medical practice. The point is simply that there is no such thing as a treatment that is "100 per cent safe." If conventional doctors are being held responsible for the occasional consequences of their therapies, then so should complementary practitioners, and they should acknowledge that the belief systems on which they rely are immensely powerful and potentially dangerous. The more honest we all are, the better for our patients.

Conclusion: A Credo

Perhaps the conclusion of this book can be expressed most easily as a personal credo. It happens to seem less clumsy when written by one of us (R.B.), although both of us share this set of beliefs and values.

Researching and writing this book has been for both of us a personal journey, and could never have been anything else. At the end of it, however, there are aspects that are even more personal for me than for Karl—influenced by my own experience as a patient, and affecting my attitude as a doctor to other patients, to illness, to treatment and to human behaviour.

I spent most of my undergraduate and early postgraduate training learning about diseases. Our medical school curriculum covered the range of human disease, and they seemed important because none of us would have graduated as doctors if we did not know enough about them. Only incidentally, as a side effect of meeting patients and only by chance or serendipity, did I learn anything about human beings. If it hadn't happened, I probably wouldn't have missed it, because at the time I did not have a burning desire to be a "people-doctor."

I made my decision to become a doctor at the age of eight and I cannot say that it was ever a true vocation or calling. I think my real reasons were slightly masochistic: medicine seemed to be difficult, arduous and demanding. At the time, I wanted to be absorbed into a formalized and circumscribed discipline, and it was only of secondary importance to me then that I would be caring for sick humans. Not all doctors are like that; many do have a genuine vocation, but it isn't a requirement for the job. Medical school interview boards ask you why you want to be a doctor, but "Because I feel called" is not deemed a good answer. Complementary practitioners, on the other hand, seem to be mostly self-selected, and that selection is often on the basis of a deep desire to help humans (although there are obviously a few charlatans). The philosophies and skills of complementary practitioners are therefore based on an understanding of (and a deeply rooted desire to understand and help) human beings—and only to a lesser extent on the understanding of diseases. That difference in emphasis initially made many of us in conventional medicine (particularly me) uneasy—first, because we spent so long learning about diseases, and second, because we may feel less competent and skilled in dealing with the human aspects of those diseases. Hence, as complementary medicine became more prominent, our initial reaction was to respond to the apparent threat by behaving defensively.

Perhaps the threat was never real. We conventional doctors feared—among other things—the possibility that complementary practitioners were claiming superior knowledge and abilities in dealing with serious disease. Some practitioners were doing that—and those claims have usually remained unproven—but most of complementary medicine is about symptoms, and not about disease. Although this may at first seem slightly cock-eyed, it makes sense when one considers that most visits to the healer are precipitated by symptoms, and that on average nearly half of those visits are not precipitated by something that we would call a true disease.

In my medical training, I didn't learn very much about the human qualities that might help me in medical practice. In those days, there was no teaching on "Interpersonal Skills" in the medical school curriculum—and that was a serious omission. I needed to learn more about how to respond to the symptoms of humans at the same time as I treated their diseases. Nowadays, things are changing. Contemporary medical students are taught far more about the human aspects of medicine, and about communication and emphatic skills than in my day. However, as a group, we conventional doctors have not yet taken this lesson fully on board, and in some respects that is why this book was necessary in the first place.

So, to come clean and confess my position, I am primarily a mechanistic doctor. Working with patients who have cancer, it would be difficult to be otherwise: the disease requires a great deal of factual knowledge in order to get the initial treatment right. But in addition to that, the impact of the disease dramatically affects every aspect of the patient's life and behaviour. Only a foolish or blindly evangelical healer would ignore that aspect—and most of us are neither of those things. Hence I accept without reservation the idea that there is something very special in the interaction between the healer—even when it's me—and the patient. To that extent I should perhaps call myself a reconstructed mechanist.

Perhaps I can explain that adjective "reconstructed" a little more fully. Four centuries ago, Descartes hypothesized that the human mind and the human body were two entirely different objects. The body was a machine, the mind a spirit. He compared the mechanics of the human body to a clock—a healthy human being was like a clock that kept good time, a sick human was like a clock that didn't work. Nowadays, the more current analogy for pure mechanists is the car. If you are an unreconstructed mechanist, you treat the human body as a car, and its doctors as garage mechanics who fix the engine without referring to the personality of the driver.

My own view—that of the reconstructed mechanist—is that if human beings are like cars, they are like a sort of Magic Car in which the characteristics of the car alter the driver, and the characteristics of the driver caused durable and structural changes in the car. Persistent fast driving causes over-development of the cylinders, over-cautious driving causes hypertrophy of the brakes and so on. I believe that we are born with certain biological characteristics, some good, some bad. We are dealt a hand of cards at birth, so to speak, and those characteristics affect our attitudes and our horizons (that's the mechanistic part of my viewpoint). Perhaps it would be a fairer world if it were otherwise, but this is the way it is. Certainly whatever hand you are dealt, there is some room for change, for some exchanging and shuffling (which is the reconstructed part of my viewpoint) but still, at the extremes, a really bad hand is a really bad hand, and a superb one is a superb one. If you happen to be born very short and of short parents, you probably won't make it as a basketball player or a British policeman. If you happen to be born with a propensity to auto-immune disease—as I was—you probably won't make a career as a professional athlete (which I haven't). That may summarize the mechanistic side of the human condition, but it is not the sum total of it. There is much more to life (and illness) than the randomness of biology.

Although I am a (liberal) mechanist as regards disease, I am also an empiricist as regards human emotions. I understand the power of empathy and the value of sympathy (as donor and recipient).

As a cancer specialist, I spend about 70 per cent of my working week looking after patients (the rest of the time is for teaching and research). Of that 70 per cent, I estimate that I spend perhaps 60 per cent of it talking and listening to my patients. The rest of that "patient-care" time I spend in examining the patients, organizing tests and X-rays and prescribing treatment. Most of the time I spend with patients, then, is taken up with talking and listening. Much of it is spent dealing with bad news and its impact on the patient and family (good news, although not infrequent, takes much less time to discuss). So, although I am a conventional doctor, conventionally trained, conventionally employed and conventionally paid, I spend over 40 per cent of my working week "just chattering." I can't necessarily *prove* that that time is valuably spent, but it is fair to say that many of my patients and their family members appreciate the time spent in dialogue, and many of them feel that it is the most important aspect of their care.

Of course, good communication alone is not enough. Conventional doctors have got to get the medical management of their patients right first. It is absolutely no use being the most communicative and empathetic doctor for miles around if you mistakenly treat a patient with a heart attack as a case of indigestion. The human aspects of medicine are added to—not substituted for—getting the medical facts straight first.

I would say that, like most cancer physicians, I spend some of my time dispensing medicine, and some of it dispensing magic—and there does not seem to be (to me at any rate) a conflict. Many of my patients do also visit complementary practitioners, usually in addition to our treatment, sometimes instead of it. I never argue with that (it would be no use even if I did) but I continue to make my own recommendations as to what conventional medicine has to offer (which, sometimes, is "no further treatment").

Perhaps cancer patients require more dialogue than patients with less serious diseases; we don't know for certain. But we do know the value of effective doctor-patient communication has been demonstrated time and time again. It may consist solely of words exchanged between individuals, but the dialogue may have tremendous value even so.

To boil it all down to a few sentences, I think I know—although I was never taught it at medical school—that doctors are not all the same and that the individual doctor makes a difference to the outcome of the same treatment. I think I know that using my own emotions as a resource and employing the communication skills that I have now acquired, I have a particular effect on my patients. I am certain that patient = person + disease.

In my view, conventional and complementary medicine need not fight each other over territorial rights, provided that both are scrupulously honest when it comes to the effect of their ministrations on disease (particularly serious disease), and both are scrupulously observant of what they are doing for the human being who brings the disease to the healer for help.

All of us—whether we are committed to conventional medicine, complementary medicine, both or neither—have to be honest. While conventional doctors still have much to learn in order to be good people-doctors and healers, complementary practitioners have to learn to be honest about their powers and about their limitations.

What we all need when we're ill

We all need more than the bare facts when we're ill. As we have stressed constantly throughout this book, medical facts are only one component of medicine. There is more to looking after a patient than simply selecting the appropriate medical fact-box, cranking the handle and churning out the correct treatment. As we've seen repeatedly, most patients want more from their doctors than the bare scientific facts; they want their doctors to be healers as well. And perhaps it is that desire that makes the difference. In fact, perhaps there are two desires involved in the patient-healer interaction—the desire of the patient to be made well, and the desire of the healer to make the patient well. Those may both be very powerful forces, capable of modifying almost any bodily symptom and the satisfaction in the outcome that both parties may feel. Perhaps, in some respects, for the non-acute and the unarguable diseases, those two desires are a major ingredient in the relationship. If the patient wants to feel better and the healer wants to make the patient feel better, then it may be less important precisely what the healer gives (or believes) provided he or she doesn't do anything to make the condition worse. Mutual expectations may profoundly affect the atmosphere of the interaction and may also dramatically change what each party thinks of the outcome.

In the final analysis, we can see quite clearly that diseases need treatment, but human beings need a healer. The healer may or may not give medicine, but in virtually every situation, he or she has to give some magic as well. Diseases need medicine, but human beings who suffer will always need a touch of magic.

NOTES

Chapter 2 The Origins of Healing

1 For a delightful overview, see C. Mettler, *The History of Medicine* (The Blakiston Company, 1947).

2 A bezoar was held by legend to be the crystallized tears of a deer that had been bitten by a snake. In fact, most bezoars used in therapy were gallstones found in the stomachs of goats. W.A. Silverman, "The Optimistic Bias Favoring Medical Attention" in *Controlled Clinical Trial* (New York: Elsevier Science, 1991).

3 Noted by H.W. Haggard and quoted in W. Silverman, *Human Experimentation* (Oxford: Oxford Medical Publications, 1985).

Chapter 3 Encounters of a Healing Kind

1 L. Payer, *Medicine and Culture* (London: Gollancz, 1990) pp. 74-84.

2 F. Beraud, *Le Foie de Francais* (Paris: Stock/Laurence Pernond, 1983).

3 R.E. Kendell, P. Pichot and M. von Cranach, "Diagnostic Criteria of English, French and German Psychiatrists," *Psychological Medicine* (4) 1974: 187-195.

4 Extract from the most important existing work on Chinese medicine, *Huang Ti Nel Ching*

5 A. Simon, D. Worthen, and J. Mitas, "An Evaluation of Iridology," *Journal of the American Medical Association* 1979

6 Reporting a discussion in which he asked the mother of a patient for consent to surgery on her son, Sir Frederick Treves recorded that the mother replied, "Oh! It is all very well to talk about consenting, but who is to pay for the funeral?" F. Treves, *The Old Receiving Room*, (London: Cassell & Co., 1923).

Chapter 4 A Taxonomy of Healing

1 It should be noted that most patients do not experience any symptoms related to relocation of the ureters—in fact, symptoms

directly and genuinely caused by the relocation would be exceptionally rare.

2 Adapted from R. Gibson, and S. Gibson, *Homeopathy for Everyone* (London: Penguin Books, 1987).

Chapter 5 Philosophical Attractions

1 "The Reharmoniser—A Practical Solution to an Unavoidable Problem." Brochure from Light Harmonics Inc., Babylon, New York.

2 H.R. Parcells, "For Better Health." Pamphlet from Parcells System of Scientific Living Inc., Albuquerque, New Mexico.

3 J. Sheridan, "The Technology of Entelev IND-20258 and Cancell an Identical Material." Brochure accompanying drug, May 1989.

4 From publicity material sent to potential patients by Dr. Hariton Alivizatos, Athens, Greece.

5 G. Naessens, "714-X—A Highly Promising Non-Toxic Treatment For Cancer and Other Immune Deficiencies." Publicity material published by author.

6 G.L. Glum, *Calling of an Angel—The True Story of René Caisse and an Indian Herbal Medicine Called Essiac, Nature's Cure for Cancer* (Los Angeles: Silent Walker Publishing, 1988).

7 From publicity material sent to potential patients by Dr. Hariton Alivizatos, Athens, Greece.

8 B. Lynes, and J. Crane, *The Cancer Cure That Worked—Fifty Years of Suppression* (Toronto: Marcus Books, 1987).

9 Health Protection Branch, Health and Welfare Canada, *714-X An Unproven Product*. Published by Health and Welfare Canada in the Issues series, January 1990.

10 C. Bird, *The Galileo of the Microscope* (St. Lambert, Quebec: Les Presses de L'Université de la Personne, 1990).

11 D. Spiegel, J.R. Bloom, H.C. Kraemer, E. Gottheil, "Effect of Psychosocial Treatment on Survival of Patients with Breast Cancer," *The Lancet* ii (1989): 888-896.

Chapter 7 Alternative Explanations of the Inexplicable

1 K. Takagi, T. Sasaki, and N. Basugi, "Spontaneous Disappearance

of Cerebellopontine Angle Arachnoid Cyst," *Neurological Surgery* 15 (1987): 295-299.

2 Y. Yamanouchi, K. Someda, and N. Oka, "Spontaneous Disappearance of Middle Fossa Arachnoid Cyst After Head Injury," *Child's Nervous System* 2 (1986): 40-43.

3 W. Boyd, *The Spontaneous Regression of Cancer* (Springfield, Ill.: Charles Thomas, 1966).

4 T.C. Everson, "Spontaneous Regression of Cancer," *Journal of the New York Academy of Sciences* 114 (1964): 721-735.

5 Dr. Paul Mueller, St. Michael's Hospital, Toronto (personal communication).

6 W.D. Rees, S.B. Dover, and T.S. Low-Beer, *British Medical Journal* 295 (August 1, 1987): 318.

7 J.A. Collins, and C.F. Snow, "Gastrointestinal Polyps" in E. Rubenstein and D.D. Federmann (eds.) *Scientific American Medicine* (New York: Scientific American, 1990, Chapter 4: XIII).

8 P. Brohn, *Gentle Giants—The Powerful Story of One Woman's Unconventional Struggle Against Cancer* (London: Century Hutchinson, 1986).

9 David Hume, *Essays and Treatises on Several Subjects*, Edinburgh 1809, p. 121.

Chapter 8 Getting Better or Feeling Better

1 Dr. Arthur Shapiro writing in the 1950s (quoted in G. Watts, *Pleasing the Patient* [London: Faber and Faber, 1992]) defined the placebo as "any therapeutic procedure (or that component of any therapeutic procedure) which is given deliberately to have an effect, or unknowingly has an effect on a patient, symptoms, syndrome or disease, but which is objectively without specific activity for the condition being treated. The therapeutic procedure may be given with or without conscious knowledge that the procedure is a placebo, may be an active (non-inert) or nonactive (inert) procedure and includes therefore all medical procedures no matter how specific—oral and parenteral (= non-oral) medication, topical (= local) preparations inhalants, and mechanical, surgical and psychological procedures. The placebo must

be differentiated from the placebo effect which may or may not occur and which may be favourable or unfavourable. The placebo effect is defined as the changes produced by placebos."

2   M. Battezatti, A. Tagliaferro, and G. de Marchi, "La Legatura Delle Due Arterie Mammarie Interne Nei Disturbi Di Vascolarizzazione Del Miocardio: Nota Preventiva Relativa Di Primi Dati: Sperimetnali E Clinic," *Minerva Medicina* 48 (1955): 1176-1188.

3   R.P. Glover, "A New Surgical Approach to the Problem of Myocardial Revascularisation in Coronary Artery Disease," *Journal of the Arkansas Medical Society* 54 (1957): 223-234.

4   D.C. Sabiston, and A. Blalock, "Experimental Ligation of Internal Mammary Artery and Its Effect on Coronary Artery Occlusion," *Surgery* 43 (1958): 906-912.

5   L.A. Cobb, G.I. Thomas, D.H. Dillard, K.A. Merendino, and R.A. Bruce, "An Evaluation of Internal-Mammary Artery Ligation by a Double-Blind Technic," *New England Journal of Medicine* 260 (1959): 1115-1118.

6   E.G. Dimond, F. Kittle, and J.E. Crockett, "Comparison of Internal Mammary Artery Ligation and Sham Operation for Angina Pectoris," *American Journal of Cardiology* (1960): 483-486.

7   H.K. Beecher, "The Powerful Placebo," *Journal of the American Medical Association* 159 (1955): 1602-1606.

8   J. Frank, "Psychotherapy of Bodily Illness: An Overview," *Psychotherapy and Psychosomatics* 26 (1975): 192-202.

9   J.D. Levine, et al., "The Mechanism of Placebo Analgaesia," *The Lancet* ii (1978): 654-657.

10 J.J.C. Smart, "Sensations and Brain Processes," *Philosophical Reviews* 68 (1959): 141-156.

11 J. Randi, *The Faith Healers* (New York: Prometheus Books, 1987).

12 B. Klopfer, "Psychological Variables in Human Cancer," *Journal of Projective Techniques* 21 (1957): 221-340.

13 L.C. Park, and L. Covi, "Nonblind Placebo Trial," *Archives of General Psychiatry* 12 (1965): 336-345.

14 R.S. Lipman, L.C. Park, and K. Rickels, "NIMH-PSC Outpatient Study of Drug-Set Interaction: II, Differential interpretation of

reliable side-effect," Research protocol 1962 (quoted in Park and Covi).

15 H. Benson, and D.P. McCallie, "Angina Pectoris and the Placebo Effect," *New England Journal of Medicine* 300 (1979): 1424-1429.

16 Socrates quoted in L.R. Kass, *Toward a More Natural Science, Biology and Human Affairs* (New York: The Free Press, 1991).

17 V.L. Gott, J.S. Donahoo, R.R. Brawley, and L.S. Griffith "Current Surgical Approaches to Ischaemic Heart Disease," *Current Problems in Surgery* (1973) 10.

18 P. Clifford, R.A. Clift, and J.K. Duff, "Nitrogen Mustard Therapy Combined with Autologous Marrow Infusion," *The Lancet* i (1961): 687-689.

19 This was one eye-catching scheme that flourished during the boom of gullibility in England known as the South-Sea Bubble. Sadly, the real name of the perpetrator is not known, so we invented Hieronymous Thompson as a John Doe *nom de plume*.

20 M. Baum, "The Treatment of Breast Cancer: Time for a Paradigm Shift," lecture, Toronto, September 1992.

21 W.A. Silverman, *Retrolental Fibroplasia: A Modern Parable* (New York: Grune and Stratton, 1980).

22 D.M. Eddy, and J.D. Billings, "The Quality of Medical Evidence and Medical Practice." Paper prepared for the National Leadership Commission on Health Care.

23 P.H. Richardson, and C.A. Vincent, "Acupuncture for the Treatment of Pain: A Review of Evaluative Research," *Pain* 24 (1986): 15-40.

24 G.T. Riet, J. Kleijnen, and P. Knipschild, "A Meta-Analysis of Studies into the Effect of Acupuncture on Addiction," *British Journal of General Practice* 40 (1990): 379-382; G.T. Riet, J. Kleijnen, and P. Knipschild, "Acupuncture and chronic pain: a criteria-based meta-analysis," 1192-1199.

25 B. Pomeranz, and G. Stux (eds.) *Scientific Bases of Acupuncture* (New York: Springer-Verlag 1989).

26 T.W. Meade, S. Dyer, W. Browne, J. Townsend, and A.O. Frank, "Low Back Pain of Mechanical Origin: Randomised Comparison of Chiropractic and Hospital Outpatient Treatment," *British Medical*

Journal 300 (1990): 1431-1437. B.W. Koes, et al., "Randomised Clinical Trial of Manipulative Therapy and Physiotherapy for Persistent Back and Neck Complaints: Results of One-Year Follow-Up," *British Medical Journal* 304 (1992): 601-605.

27 B. Inglis, and R. West, *The Alternative Health Guide* (London: Michael Joseph 1983).

28 M.P. Sheehan, and D.J. Atheron, "A Controlled Trial of Traditional Chinese Medicinal Plants in Widespread Non-Exudative Atopic Eczema," *British Journal of Dermatology* 126 (1992): 179-184.

29 J. Kleijnen, P. Knipschild, and G.T. Riet, "Clinical Trials of Homeopathy," *British Medical Journal* 302 (1991): 316-323.

30 GRECHO (Group de Recherches et d'Essais Cliniques en Homéopathie), "Evaluation de deux produits homéopathique sur la reprise du transit après chirugie digestive," *Presse Médicale* 18 (1989): 59-62.

31 B. Brigo, and G. Serpelloni, "Homeopathic Treatment of Migraine: A Randomized Double-Blind Controlled Study of Sixty Cases," *Berlin Journal on Research in Homeopathy* 1 (1991): 98-106.

32 Although we filmed the data-analysis of this study, in deference to the investigators we have agreed not to publish full details of the study until the publication of the full results of the trial in a medical journal.

33 R.G. Gibson, S.L.M. Gibson, A.D. MacNeill, and W.W. Buchanan, "Homeopathic Therapy in Rheumatoid Arthritis: Evaluation by Double-Blind Clinical Therapeutic Trial," *British Journal of Clinical Pharmacology* 9 (1980): 453-259.

34 D.T. Reilly, M.A. Taylor, C. McSharry, and T. Aitchison, "Is Homeopathy a Placebo Response: Controlled Trial of Homeopathic Potency with Pollen in Hayfever as a Model," *The Lancet* ii (1986): 881-886.

35 J. Randi, *The Faith Healers* (New York: Prometheus Books, 1987).

36 P. Brohn, *Cancer Help Centre: Cancer and Its Non-Toxic Treatment* (Bristol: Bristol Cancer Help Centre, 1985).

37 F.S. Bagenal, D.F. Easton, E. Harris, C.E.D. Chilvers, and T.J. McElwain, "Survival of Patients with Breast Cancer Attending

Bristol Cancer Help Centre," *The Lancet* ii (1990): 606–610.

38 C.E.D. Chilvers, D.F. Easton, F.S. Bagenal, E. Harris, and T.J. McElwain, letter in *The Lancet* ii (1990): 1886–1888.

39 W. Bodmer, letter in *The Lancet* ii (1990): 1188.

40 C.E.D. Chilvers, D.F. Easton, F.S. Bagenal, E. Harris, and T.J. McElwain, letter in *The Lancet* ii (1990): 1886–1888.

41 B.S. Siegel, *Love, Medicine and Miracles—Lessons Learned About Self-Healing from a Surgeon's Experience with Exceptional Patients* (New York: Harper and Row, 1986).

42 B.S. Siegel, Peace, *Love and Healing—Body-Mind Communication and the Path to Self-Healing: An Exploration* (New York: Harper and Row, 1989).

43 H. Morganstern, G.A. Gellert, S.D. Walter, A.M. Ostfeld, and B.S. Siegel, "The Impact of a Psychosocial Support Program on Survival with Breast Cancer," *Journal of Chronic Disease* 37 (1984): 273–

44 D. Spiegel, J.R. Bloom, and I. Yalom, "Group Support for Patients with Metastatic Cancer," *Archives of General Psychiatry* 38 (1981): 527–533.

45 D. Spiegel, J.R. Bloom, H. Kraemer, and E. Gottheil, "Effect of Psychosocial Treatment on Survival of Patients with Metastatic Breast Cancer," *The Lancet* ii (1989): 888–891.

46 L.C. Park, and L. Covi, "Nonblind Placebo Trial," *Archives of General Psychiatry* 12 (1965): 336–345.

Chapter 9 Synthesis: Magic and Medicine

1 "The heaviest guard is placed at the gateway to nothing…because the state of emptiness is too shameful to be revealed." F. Scott Fitzgerald, *Tender Is the Night.*

2 *Emotional Factors in the Pathogenesis of Tuberculosis*

3 B.R. Cassileth, et al., "Survival and Quality of Life Among Patients Receiving Unproven as Compared with Conventional Cancer Therapy," *New England Journal of Medicine* 324 (1991): 1180–1185.

4 D. Roter (study from the Toronto Conference).

5 J.W. Eisele, and D.T. Resy, "Deaths Related to Coffee Enemas," *Journal of the American Medical Association* 244 (1980): 1608–1609.

6   G.A. Curt, "Warning on Immunoaugmentative Therapy," *New England Journal of Medicine* 246 (1984): 714-715.

7   (Anon.) "Isolation of Human T-lymphotropic Virus Type III/Lymphadenopathy-Associated Virus from Serum Proteins Given to Cancer Patients," *Leads from the Morbidity and Mortality Weekly Reports* 254 (1985): 1139.

8   *The Health Service Journal*, October 25, 1990, p. 1600.

9   R. Buckman, *How To Break Bad News* (London: Macmillan Medical, 1993).

INDEX